To b

May ',

Filled with endless

hugs and kisses

and More Love than

you'll know how to

handle. All
    May your dreams
Come true —

        Love
J Knuth i Deb

The Prescription for a Happy and Healthy Child

113 Questions Answered by a Top Pediatrician (Ages 0–5)

Dr. Daniela Atanassova-Lineva, M.D.

Dr. Shellie Hipsky, Ed.D.

Aurora Corialis Publishing

Pittsburgh, PA

The Prescription for a Happy and Healthy Child: 113 Questions
Answered by a Top Pediatrician (Ages 0–5)

For more information, please email the publisher
cori@auroracorialispublishing.com.

Paperback ISBN: 978-1-958481-04-2

EBook ISBN: 978-1-958481-05-9

Printed in the United States of America

Cover by Karen Captline, BetterBe Creative

Edited by Renee Picard, Aurora Corialis Publishing

DISCLAIMER

The information in the book *The Prescription for a Happy and Healthy Child* is true and complete to the best of our knowledge at the time of publishing. The content of this book is for informational purposes only and is not intended to diagnose, treat, cure, or prevent any condition or disease. This is not to conflict with or replace in any way advice from your own pediatrician. The advice and strategies found within may not be suitable for every situation. There are no promises or guarantees that this book will have the information you need. It does not serve as a medical diagnostic tool. The authors and publishers disclaim all liability in connection with this book's information and its use.

Although the publisher and the authors have made every effort to ensure that the information in this book was correct at press time and while this publication is designed to provide accurate information in regard to the subject matter covered, the publisher and the authors assume no responsibility for errors, inaccuracies, omissions, or any other inconsistencies herein and hereby disclaim any liability to any party for any loss, damage, or disruption caused by errors or omissions, whether such errors or omissions result from negligence, accident, or any other cause.

Use of this book implies your acceptance of these disclaimers.

DEDICATION

This book is dedicated to our wonderful children:

Dr. Daniela Atanassova-Lineva's Stefani and Daniel & Dr. Shellie Hipsky's Alyssa and Jacob

PLUS, we dedicate this book to the Children of the World!

ADVANCE PRAISE FOR THE PRESCRIPTION FOR A HAPPY AND HEALTHY CHILD

"As a psychologist and stress expert on children, I would offer that Dr. Daniela's book is extremely comprehensive, offering solutions and information on almost every topic concerning children and their development. With Dr. Shellie's added experiences as a parent, lending expertise and warmth, *The Prescription for a Happy and Healthy Child* is the new guidebook for bringing up the next generation. Together they bring a mix of advice and resources that will change the lives of parents and their children."

~ Nancy Mramor, Ph.D.

"This book provides excellent information from one of the best pediatricians in New York City. I'm sure it will help millions of parents with all the difficult questions that come with raising a child. As a physician and a father of three, I'm glad this book is available because it has all the information you need to know about caring for your children."

~ Dr. Nayaz Ahmed, M.D., Pediatrician and Primary Care Physician at NY Health + Hospitals

"As a Nurse Practitioner, I believe that empowerment is key to health and well-being. Authors Dr. Shellie Hipsky and Dr. Daniela Atanassova-Lineva have done an excellent job of empowering parents by sharing their knowledge and expertise and giving a blueprint of care that is easy to understand."

~ Teresa Palmer, Nurse Practitioner and Bestselling Author

"This book is wonderful! I would have loved to have it handy during my child's early years. It is an impressive and thorough collection of researched and practical advice for parents, grandparents, and caregivers. It is everything you need to know to help you care for your child ages 0–5. Particularly helpful were the author's personalization of strategies to manage behaviors and emotions in your child. As a health care provider and parent, this is the exact prescription you want to fill!"

~ Mary E. Ciesa, Adult Nurse Practitioner and Maternal Child Clinical Nurse Specialist

"Wow! What a gift to have one book that is the go-to for parenthood questions with a wide array of topics. This book literally covers everything that new parents need, and as a mother of six children, I am highly recommending this book!"

~ Marta Sauret Greca, Bestselling Author and CEO of Media - The Creative Agency

"I highly recommend that every parent read *The Prescription for a Happy and Healthy Child*! I was in awe of the level of detail and subjects covered by Dr. Daniela Atanassova-Lineva and Dr. Shellie Hipsky in this book. When two amazing mommies who are well respected in their own fields combine their expertise and share their experience with the world, it creates an absolutely invaluable resource. As a mother and doctor myself, I really wish I would had this book when I had my daughter 8 years ago. I've also seen the special bond that Dr. Shellie has with her own two amazing children and her mother, which makes this collaboration with respected pediatrician Dr. Daniela an even more meaningful book.

~ Dr. Hoa Nguyen, Optometrist Specializing in Pediatric Eye Care

"The Prescription for a Happy and Healthy Child is a must-have guidebook for parents from birth through 5 years old. Now as a parent and grandparent, I found up-to-date answers to the most common questions that I had as a new parent, including choosing a pediatrician, crying babies, diaper rash, potty training, injuries and illnesses, special needs, child safety, and much more. The book offers a practical balance between real-life parenting experiences from Dr. Shellie Hipsky, Ed.D., and clinical professional medical advice from Dr. Daniela Atanassova-Lineva, M.D."

~ Sabrina Protic, Bestselling Author & Financial Coach with the World Class Partners Foundation

"This book is a must read for anyone raising young children! As a parent of 3 kids, I am very impressed with Dr. Daniela's medical knowledge, as well as Dr. Shellie's authentic sharing of her challenges in raising her children. As a busy healthcare professional, I see tremendous value in the information presented; it's to the point, descriptive, and diagnostic. The authors go beyond giving great information. They share the frustration and worries of the parents, whether it is about a rash or an episode of depression! This is truly a practical handbook of modern parenting."

~ Dr. Emily Letran, DDS, MS, CHPC, Family Dentist and International Speaker on Parenting

"As a founder in the digital healthcare sector, I highly recommend *The Prescription for a Happy and Healthy Child*. Dr. Daniela Atanassova-Lineva and Dr. Shellie Hipsky have crafted a comprehensive guide that addresses the most pressing questions parents have about their children's health. The book is written in an accessible and easy-to-understand format, and provides practical tips and insights that will benefit both new and experienced parents. It's a valuable resource for anyone seeking to raise happy, healthy children."

~ Sara Makin, MS.Ed., L.P.C., N.C.C., Founder and CEO of Makin Wellness Online Therapy and Counseling

"This is one of the most amazing books for parents. Through it, you can learn how to raise a happy and healthy kid. I am a mother of a son who is autistic and nonverbal. I also work with children with disabilities every day. I suggest that everyone make sure that they read this helpful and informative book!"

~ Shangwe Mgaya, Director and Founder of Living Together Autistic Foundation (Li-TAFO) in Tanzania, Africa

"This clearly written book is a great help for parents who have babies and young children to know what to do in any situation. It is very accessible and understandable for all people to read, even if they are not from the United States.

Parents can find a lot of practical knowledge in this book."

~ Alla Shalomova, Head Nurse at Junction Clinic Pediatrics

"My husband and I were newly assigned to an overseas military base when I was 8-months pregnant. No family. No friends. No clue of what to expect as new parents. We relied on medical books to guide us. This no-nonsense book with both practical application and stories is exactly what we needed in our lives as new parents navigating foreign territory. The guidance of Drs. Shellie and Daniela will help countless parents internationally."

~ Dr. Michelle Mras, Ph.D., "The Parent Compass," International Speaker, and Bestselling Author

"When my first daughter was two months old, I moved to a new city. I had no family, no friends, no church home ... I was literally starting all over. I wish I had the guidance this book provides for asking questions to a new pediatrician to take the anxiety and stress out of figuring out what I needed to know before making the choice. I was blessed with an amazing pediatrician, but this book provides a roadmap of discovery for new parents. Thank you to Dr. Shellie and Dr. Daniela for adding to the credible and useful resources parents really need."

~ Dr. Jessica Merritt, Ph.D., President of the Care Based Leadership Collaborative

ACKNOWLEDGEMENTS

Special thank yous to those who made this book possible. Cori Wamsley at Aurora Corialis Publishing did a dynamite job of getting this parenting book to press and beyond. Karen Captline created the beautiful cover of this book. Kelli Komondor and Charissa Lauren have helped us spread the good word through PR and marketing to the parents of the world about *The Prescription for a Happy and Healthy Child.* Thank you also to Ani Marie Mariotti for helping behind the scenes with Dr. Daniela and Dr. Shellie on our quest to support parents internationally to raise happy and healthy children. Many thanks to Dr. Nataly Apollonsky, MD, who did a wonderful job with the foreword from the perspective of a pediatrician and mother! Thank you to Dr. Daniela's patients and their parents for being featured in this book.

Finally, a special thank you to you, the parent or caregiver who is reading this book. We greatly appreciate you and we hope that you will write a positive review of *The Prescription for a Happy and Healthy Child* on Amazon or Barnes and Noble online.

FOREWORD

Dr. Nataly Apollonsky, MD,

Chief of Pediatric Hematology at St. Christopher's Hospital for Children

I recall meeting Dr. Daniela Atanassova-Lineva during the first week of our residency at the Mount Sinai Pediatrics affiliated Elmhurst Hospital in Queens. First weeks are often hard. New residents are trying to quickly learn on the job and to get to know each other. Dr. Daniela made it easy for everyone around her. She was always so warm, open, and supportive. I felt she had such great energy. Working with her was a pleasure because she is very reliable, knowledgeable, and confident. She has always been a person to go to if you need support or a second opinion when making important decisions.

There were many similarities in our pediatric journeys.

She was an immigrant like me. I had completed my medical education back in Russia. Dr. Daniela was from Bulgaria. Neither of us spoke English well and we had our residency at Mount Sinai together. Dr. Daniela actually learned English while she was taking the Kaplan Medical course to pass the exams in the states. We were learning the language while we were completing our residencies.

And we were both mothers. At that time, I had come to America with my two small children from St. Petersburg, Russia, and Dr. Daniela had come from Bulgaria with her baby Stefani, who was one year old at the time. As new mothers with young children, working in a country far from where we were raised, we had questions.

Even with my extensive medical background, I wish that I would have had a book like *The Prescription for a Happy and Healthy Child* when questions with my own family arose because, no matter how knowledgeable you are—as a new mother—you are always seeking out the vital answers to meet the needs of your children.

My medical journey was successful. After finishing my pediatric residency I decided to focus on pediatric hematology and oncology and completed fellowship training. Currently I am a section chief of Hematology in Children's Hospital. Working with children and helping sick kids is more than a job, it is my passion, and I greatly enjoy it.

Dr. Daniela went on to run her own successful pediatric practice in Queens, New York, for the last 13 years. She is board certified in pediatrics and is a member of several prominent medical organizations. She has a busy office and sees a lot of patients every day, but she always makes sure that she spends enough time with the families and tries to answer all the questions.

The parents of Dr. Daniela's patients rave online with five stars and comments like:

"We always get excellent and reliable service from Dr. Daniela."

"Dr. Daniela is an incredible doctor!"

"I'd like to express my sincere appreciation for the professional care given by Dr. Daniela and her staff. She's amazing! Her ability to diagnose and communicate your medical needs is second to none."

I am a proud mother of four. My children's ages are 14, 16, 27, and 30 years of age. I absolutely would have trusted Dr. Daniela as my children's doctor when they were young!

Dr. Daniela treats all of her pediatric patients as if they were her own children. Through this book, she wants to help the children of the world by helping parents answer their most common questions.

Dr. Daniela Atanassova-Lineva has successfully teamed up with Dr. Shellie Hipsky. Dr. Shellie is the CEO of Inspiring Lives International, the executive director of the Global Sisterhood nonprofit that helps women and children around the world, and she has written 15 international bestselling books. Most importantly for this project, she was a tenured university education professor. Dr. Shellie co-authored this book with Dr. Daniela in a style that will teach you. You will learn what to do to support your children from birth to age five—whether you're dealing with a common illness or an unexpected emergency—so you can be proactive instead of reactive.

I highly recommend *The Prescription for a Happy and Healthy Child* to you so you can be the best parent you can be while keeping your child safe and well. I personally wanted to support this book because I believe in the power of knowledge. I trust that you will learn from Dr. Daniela's 113 responses to the important questions that she answers daily from parents. In this noisy, busy world of media and tons of information, this resource will serve as an invaluable and impactful parenting guide from a doctor you can trust.

TABLE OF CONTENTS

Chapter Two: Development and Growth.. 89

INTRODUCTION: EXPECTANT PARENT

Dr. Shellie's Mom Memories as an Expectant Parent

My mother was walking outside with my son Jacob. Jacob is a Pokémon lover, who enjoys walks in nature, gravitates toward computers, loves to create with wood in his grandfather's workshop, and knows many fascinating facts. He also happens to be diagnosed with ADHD and is on the autism spectrum.

A middle schooler at the time, he asked my mom, "What is one of your favorite memories from your lifetime?" She explained that one of the most important moments was being present at the births of Jacob and his older sister Alyssa. As they walked in the sunshine outside my parents' independent living community, she told him that being a part of those precious moments with them as they entered the world was so beautiful. She exclaimed, "I was just so proud of your mom!"

When they were telling me about this bonding conversation, I was flooded with so many memories and emotions: good, terrifying, nerve-racking, and beautiful. Both of my children were ten-pound babies with big brown eyes, yet they were unique individuals from the moment they were born.

Alyssa's birth was exhausting and yet perfectly wonderful. I recall that, when they placed her on my chest, I exclaimed that she was, "So pretty. And, oh my goodness, she looks very intelligent!" Sixteen years later, that motherly instinct rings true as she is preparing for a future medical career and wows us with how creative and smart she is.

Jacob had a bit rougher entry into the world. I had a scare during my pregnancy and thought I might lose him. Then after a more difficult labor, he was born with the umbilical cord around his neck. And strangely, his first cry sounded like a noise a pterodactyl would make. Because his cry was so usual, the doctor needed to put him under anesthesia to scope his throat with a tiny camera to see what was wrong. They were worried that they may need to do a tracheotomy because they thought that his vocal cords were paralyzed.

As a former special education teacher, assistant principal of a school for special needs, and a tenured special education professor for a decade, the knowledge of what could be if he was severely disabled was very real for me. Jacob stayed in the NICU, and they let me "nest in" at the hospital to stay near my breastfeeding baby. My toddler visited her new baby brother and me there at the hospital while I prayed and tried my hardest to be the best parent I could be. We survived it. And Jacob now is expressive verbally; he grew up intelligent and tall, and he makes me so proud.

Yet, when I think back to those moments that my mom saw as the most amazing in her over seven decades on this earth, I can't help but also recall the rougher moments. I think of the exhaustion of finally bringing home my baby with

3

a loud heart monitor on— while raising a curious toddler—and writing a college educational textbook for future teachers during their nap times. The sleepless teary-eyed nights with leaking nipples and a squishy belly. Wondering if I'd ever be back to myself. And if I could really be the mother I felt my children deserved.

This was my reality as a new mother. I recall having so many questions those first 5 years of both of my children's lives as I stepped into the role of being The Mom. And that is exactly why I felt that this book with Dr. Daniela Atanassova-Lineva needed to be written for you, the new parent. Through the pages of our book you will be able to turn to one of the top pediatricians in the world, according to the professional organization International Association for Top Professionals (IATOP).

You deserve to have your important questions answered or to know where to find help when you are worried and you need a trusted expert. We compiled the most frequently asked questions gathered from Dr. Daniela's thousands of patients' parents about their children. From what

4

to do if your child gets sick or accidentally hurt—
to how to set them up for social and emotional
success—it's in The Prescription for a Happy and
Healthy Child. *Dr. Daniela has been in practice for
over twenty years in New York City. As a*

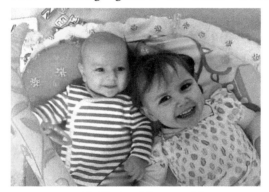

*pediatrician,
she has
heard and
responded to
countless
parenting
questions.*

*We hope
that this can
be a go-to*

Dr. Shellie's Kids as Babies

*resource for you as a parent navigating unknown
territory. You can do this! Just remember to be
kind to yourself during these balancing years.
Treat your child as an individual with unique
needs. Show them your love. We all want to have
happy and healthy children, and this can start
with the knowledge that you are gaining from
reading this book!*

Dr. Daniela's Pediatric Prescription for Expectant Parents

I am not just a pediatrician who has had a successful practice working with diverse children from all over the world in Queens, New York City. I am also a mom who loves her two children and had

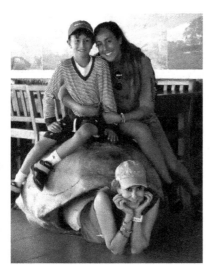

Dr. Daniela with Her Children

her own questions when my little ones were growing up. I think that this book is different from anything else you will read because I was able to capture the 113 most common questions that I have been asked during my over 20-year career and respond to them from the perspective of being a loving mother and a dedicated doctor. I have so much experience caring about both the children in my home and in my pediatric office!

Dr. Shellie Hipsky is a world-class educator, and we combine her skills with mine as a medical doctor in this book, committing to helping you have a successful first 5 years and beyond with your baby. As she helps with

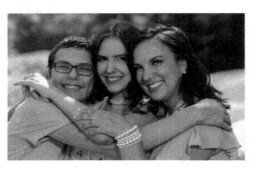

Dr. Shellie with Her Children

the education component in the book, I will home in on the medical facts and instructions you need to support your child. We are both moms who love their children!

Step One for New Parents: Finding the Right Pediatrician for Your Family

Where do we start? First, you need to find the right pediatrician for your child. Make sure that you check out your local doctor on the internet or ask other parents who live near you. Search for what others have to say about your chosen doctor. Valid places to look at are Zocdoc Reviews, Google, Facebook, Patient Pop, Yelp, and many more. Sadly, some doctors pay for their reviews, but out of hundreds more than 70% would be telling you the

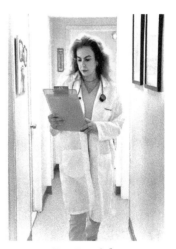

Dr. Daniela

truth. Legitimate patients are asked for their feedback only after the visit has been completed. Here are some of the important questions you could ask when interviewing to determine your child's ideal pediatric office.

Questions to Ask Your Future Pediatrician

How many years of experience and what type of experience does the pediatrician have?

Experience and exposure are crucial for a pediatrician and any doctor. The formula is simple: The more patients you treat and follow up with on their illnesses, the more experience and confidence you build. If your pediatrician tells you that they have had clinical and ER experience, this is your best bet!

What happens if the office is closed and my child needs care? Who will answer the calls? Do they have an answering service? Where do the phone calls get redirected?

After all, the last thing you want is to be left hanging when you need your doctor's advice the most.

Is the pediatrician involved with teaching?

Teaching is the best way that a doctor can stay up-to-date with the latest medical practices.

Ask yourself when you enter the office: Is it clean? Is it kid-friendly? Who is sitting behind the desk? Are they polite and knowledgeable?

Most of the time you will be communicating through the front desk employees.

How are the visits grouped? For example, ask your pediatrician if they have separate days and hours of seeing newborns, or whether the sick walk-ins are separated from well child visits.[1]

What is the average turnover time after the patient comes into the office lobby until the office visit is complete?

---

[1] A well child visit (or "well baby" visit for those under age 2) is a routine preventative health check with a pediatrician. For children under 2, those visits may be every few weeks or months. For those over 2, they are annual.

Does the office work with lactation specialists for nursing moms?

What is the pediatrician's belief regarding vaccines?

Does their office have a mobile app where you can view your chart, track the vaccines records, and follow the growth of your child?

Do they provide tele-visits?

Who are the other providers in the office?

Do they work with nurse practitioners and how does the doctor supervise them?

What should a parent do if their child gets sick during the night, weekends, or holidays?

What is the pediatrician's take on breastfeeding? For how long? How much/often? And what are the benefits?

What is your doctor's personality? Are they personable and approachable? Do they show signs of empathy and care?

Does the pediatrician support home births? The American Academy of Pediatrics (AAP) does not recommend home birth in developed countries, because of increased risk of neonatal mortality. If the parents are committed to it and follow cultural and religious beliefs, they should be educated by their pediatrician on what must be done. Such as:

- Eye care prophylaxis to prevent gonococcal conjunctivitis
- Hepatitis B and vitamin K prophylaxis
- Feeding assessment and education on latching and burping techniques
- Blood screening for hyperbilirubinemia, hearing test, oxygen pulse oximetry to assure the baby does not suffer any congenital heart diseases, and newborn screening test

It's important to note whether the pediatrician inquires about genetic tree and history of family chronic diseases. Challenge the pediatrician with questions like, "Should I collect stem cells from the umbilical cord or placenta? Which one is better, and what is the difference?"

Choosing the right pediatrician is an important step toward your child being healthy in the future. You need to feel secure in your current decision, but remember that if you need to switch pediatricians down the road, you can do that. We want this book to serve as a valuable resource. While it won't replace a doctor's care, it will help you with the most commonly asked questions by other parents like you!

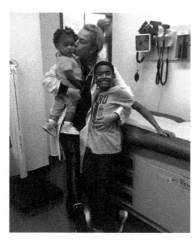

Dr. Daniela with Kids in Her Office

CHAPTER ONE: YOUR NEWBORN COMES HOME

Dr. Shellie's Mom Memories when her Newborns Came Home

I felt like I was in a haze of hormonal and sleep-deprived exhaustion after we got the baby home from the hospital. Of course, I simply adored the baby snuggles. There were moments when I would stare at my sleeping child, flooded with emotions thinking, "Wow, I made that beautiful baby?"

Yet, trying to get my baby to stop crying— trying to meet their around-the-clock newborn needs—while my own body was healing was, simply put, a lot! I was trying to figure out how to breastfeed 8 to 12 times a day, because a newborn's stomach is only the size of a ping pong ball. I was charting what was in the baby's diaper (from color to the amount of poop) to prepare for the initial well baby appointments with the pediatrician. I was learning how to be a parent to my baby as I went along, while covered in spit up and running on zero sleep. I wanted to know how to best care for my newborn. How do I deal with the umbilical cord stump? When a diaper rash flares up, how should I treat it?

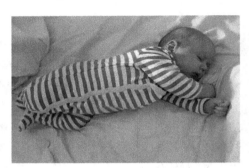

Dr. Shellie's Son as a Newborn

The newborn stage is a short period of time during the first two months of a baby's life, and it's often a combination of an emotional rollercoaster, extreme fatigue, and happiness. Many questions arise, as you'll see in this chapter!

Dr. Daniela's Pediatric Prescription for When the Newborn Comes Home

1. What should I do if my baby failed the hearing test in the hospital?

All newborns have a screening test prior to discharge from the hospital. Approximately 1–3 out of 1,000 babies fail the first hearing test. There can also be false positive results, and the most common reason for that is amniotic fluid in the middle of the ear. If your baby fails the hearing test your pediatrician will follow up with an ear, nose, and throat (ENT) doctor, or you will have a scheduled follow up at the hospital where the baby was born.

Failing to detect hearing loss may affect your baby's speech, cognitive functions, school performance, and social skills. In many countries around the world, the hearing test is not done routinely after delivery. Paying close attention to your newborn's reactions to loud noises like slamming doors, music, and loud speech is important. Any concerns should be addressed and shared with your pediatrician.

2. When does the umbilical stump fall off? And how do I take care of it?

The umbilical cord is a vascular "tube" containing two arteries and one vein that carry nutrients and oxygen to the embryo from the placenta during pregnancy. At the time of delivery, the umbilical cord is clamped (which is when it is bound by a clip to interrupt blood flow from the placenta to the fetus) or cut by using a sterile blade or scissors. Infections are rare unless there is an overgrowth of bacteria transmitted to the newborn baby from the maternal vaginal flora during vaginal delivery. If there is one artery (an SUA or single umbilical artery), the pediatrician in the delivery room might need to do additional studies to ensure your child is healthy. Some oozing from the umbilical stump in the first days of life is expected, but keeping it clean and dry is important.

There is no need to use alcohol, water, soap, or chlorhexidine, because this can delay the separation of the stump. On average, the umbilical stump will fall off in 7 to 10 days, even though up to 3 weeks is still an expected time period. To prevent the stump from getting wet with urine or from excessive rubbing, fold the diaper to lay under the cord.

If the umbilical stump does not separate by 3 weeks of age, contact your pediatrician, as some rare immune deficiencies, (like leukocyte adhesion

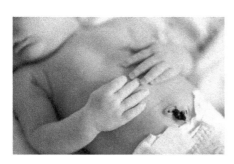

Umbilical Cord Stump

deficiency) could be a possible cause. If the umbilical stump is bleeding or you notice foul-smelling, yellowish discharge, contact your pediatrician immediately.

Umbilical cord stumps can seem perplexing for some new parents; yet, it's such a beautiful way for a baby to receive life-sustaining nutrients while inside the mother, and it should simply fall off naturally.

3. What can I do if my baby's sonogram showed water in his kidneys and they are enlarged?

Do you recall the magical day when you heard the heartbeat of your baby for the first time? This usually happens around the 15th week of pregnancy. Doppler sonograms are used to scan for anatomical anomalies, bone defects, and the baby's blood flow and circulation. Hydronephrosis (water in the kidney) may be discovered and diagnosed during routine prenatal visits by sonogram evaluation.

Always carry your discharge papers and imaging studies and present them to your new primary care physician or nurse practitioner. Fortunately, most cases are mild to moderate and if there is no underlying condition, they resolve completely by approximately 18 months of age. The kidney specialist who takes care of this condition is called a "nephrologist" or "renal doctor," and your pediatrician may refer you to one.

4. What should I know if my baby was in a breech position during my pregnancy?

"Breech position" means that your baby is laying bottom or feet first in the womb. If by the 36th week of gestation your baby is in a breech position, your obstetrician will discuss what would be the safest method of delivery. This can happen during any pregnancy, but it is more common in pregnancies with multiples, embryos with underlying congenital diseases, an abnormally shaped mother's uterus, uterine fibroids, or if there is too little or too much amniotic fluid and not enough space for the embryo. The breech position may require a C-section (cesarean birth), but regardless of the method of delivery, your baby will require a follow-up hip sonogram to rule out hip dysplasia. Breech position in the third trimester is the biggest single risk factor for hip dysplasia. The hip joint is made out of a ball (femur) and a socket (acetabulum) joint. In hip dysplasia, the ball slips in and out of the acetabulum.

By 6 weeks of age, a mandatory sonogram of the hips will be ordered by your pediatrician if your baby was breech. The imaging studies may be ordered sooner if your doctor finds clinical signs of hip dysplasia during the physical examination. The sooner the condition is discovered, addressed, and treated, the better the outcome.

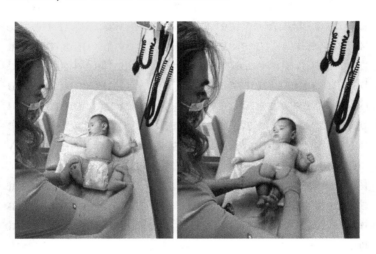

Dr. Daniela Performing the Barlow Maneuver to Rule out Hip Dysplasia

*Note: These maneuvers must be done without a diaper.

In mild cases, a "wait and watch" approach may be advised. In moderate to severe cases, harness splints (the Pavlik harness is the most thoroughly studied device for this) are used for several months. Your child will be under the care of a pediatric orthopedic surgeon for this condition.

5. Why was my baby born with a cleft lip and cleft palate? What can be done to help?

With routine prenatal care, the soft facial tissues of the fetus can be seen by week 12 of pregnancy. In a baby without a cleft lip or palate, lip closure occurs at 35 days post conception, and the fusion of the palate occurs around 56 days after birth. Cleft lips and/or cleft palates have many different causes. Gene-to-gene and gene-to-environment factors, smoking, poorly controlled diabetes, obesity, and certain anti-seizure medications have been proven to increase the risks for these conditions. Most cleft lips/palates are not associated with genetic syndromes but are rather an isolated finding.

The main challenges for babies with these conditions after birth are related to breathing and feeding. Babies with cleft palates will struggle to maintain negative pressure during latching or bottle feedings. There are special squeezable bottles and orthodontic pacifiers to support the lip and palate during soothing and feedings that help.

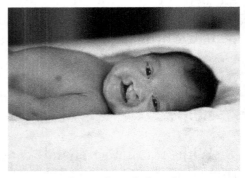

Baby with a Cleft Palate

The first reconstructive surgery could be done as early as 6 to 9 months after birth. A team that is composed of an oral maxillofacial surgeon, lactation specialist, speech therapist, and ENT doctors work together to successfully manage this craniofacial defect. In rare cases, cleft palates go unnoticed after birth. If you notice difficulties during latching and bottle feedings like choking, sneezing after feedings, drooling, or milk spilling after feedings please address it with your pediatrician.

6. Why is my baby's skin yellowish?

Every newborn baby gets their bilirubin levels checked. I often get challenged by parents to explain all possible causes for the yellowish-tinted skin. Bilirubin is a breakdown product of the red blood cells, and in newborns the life span of these cells is only 85 days compared to 120 days in adults. Because of the fast turnover, newborns produce more bilirubin than they can handle and excrete. Bilirubin is removed by the liver, which in babies is still immature, and then excreted from the body by the stool and urine.

Every newborn gets their bilirubin levels checked 24–48 hours after birth. In a baby with jaundice, the white parts of the eyes (sclera) get yellow, and the skin of the face, trunk, back, and arms gets a yellowish tint as well. If you apply pressure with your finger on the skin and quickly remove it, the skin will still remain yellow. The poop and urine of your baby will be orangey in color.

"Jaundice" is the diagnosis your doctor will use for your baby when they have a yellow hue to their skin. Depending on the baby's blood bilirubin levels, the doctor will determine if therapy is needed. Light therapy, known as "phototherapy," uses a blue-green light or light blanket to reduce the bilirubin levels. If your baby is dehydrated and has less than 4 wet diapers in 24 hours, you increase the risks for jaundice. Breast-fed babies also can have prolonged jaundice, lasting as long as 4–6 weeks, and this is the most common cause of physiological jaundice. Physiological jaundice refers to neonatal jaundice which is "normal" and clears up on its own; pathological jaundice means that there is an underlying issue and the jaundice is an illness.

If the mother and baby have different blood types, the baby may be at risk for pathological jaundice. There are rare genetic diseases and liver diseases that can be the reason for jaundice extending over the period of 2 months, and this is when immediate medical attention is mandated.

Even though most cases of "yellow baby" are due to immaturity and breastfeeding, you do not want to wait too long before you consult with your pediatrician to avoid a serious condition called "kernicterus," a type of brain damage (caused by very high levels of bilirubin) that can lead to cerebral palsy, hearing and vision loss, and intellectual and learning disabilities. Fortunately, jaundice can be caught early; plus, it is typically short-term and treatable by a medical professional, or it resolves itself within days to weeks.

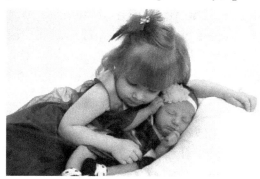
Baby with Jaundice

7. How do I heal my baby's diaper rash?

Diaper rashes, also known as "diaper dermatitis," "napkin dermatitis," or "nappy rash," are common sources of skin inflammation in infants and toddlers. The areas typically affected are the buttocks, inguinal (groin) areas, lower abdomen, and genitals. The constant friction of the diaper with the skin with the addition of moisture and increased pH (a measure of how acidic or basic a substance or solution is) are all factors contributing to the disruption of the skin barrier function. The skin's upper layer has an optimally acidic pH to maintain the skin barrier and its antibacterial defense. The presence of urinary and fecal waste in the diaper changes the pH and shifts it toward being more alkaline, which makes the skin susceptible to damage and bacterial or fungal overgrowth.

The primary irritants of the diaper area skin are urine and stool. Rarely, the diaper itself could be an irritant and causes contact dermatitis. In the latter case, other brands, including hypoallergenic options, could be considered. Some of the risk factors for diaper dermatitis are infrequent diaper changes, diarrhea, and the recent use of antibiotics. Breastfed infants have less frequent diaper rashes, and one of the theories behind this is the low stool pH in breastfed babies compared to formula-fed infants.

The most common diaper rash in infants is candida or fungal rash with the typical presentation of red beefy skin inflammation, not sparing the groin area (inguinal folds). Secondary bacterial infections are also common, including *Staphylococcus aureus* and more rarely streptococcal perianal dermatitis (the area around the anus).

There are different treatments for diaper rash. Your pediatrician will decide what topical creams or ointments to prescribe based on the clinical findings. Infants with diaper rash will present with irritability and fussiness and will have disturbed and superficial sleep due to itchiness and pain.

Baby with Candidal Diaper Rash

Preventing diaper rash by using pastes and ointments to create a more effective skin barrier is the best approach. The most commonly used ones are petrolatum, zinc oxide, or both. Frequent diaper changes, good hygiene, and daily baths will help with diaper rash prevention.

Initiating potty training at around 24 to 30 months of age, and slowly transitioning the child from using diapers to using the toilet, will help prevent diaper rashes in your toddlers.

8. Why is my baby's head flat on one side?

Don't be surprised if as a new parent you are focusing on every single detail of the physical appearance of your baby. If you notice that parts of the head appear flatter and asymmetrical, bring it to the attention of your doctor at the next well baby visit. The flattening of the head and some of the skull bones of your newborn baby can occur due to the supine (back) position that is required to keep your baby safe and prevent sudden infant death syndrome (SIDS).

Some babies are born with an asymmetric skull shape if there is less space in the womb. This can happen if they are born prematurely or their head was resting against the mother's pelvic bones or a sibling's bone in the case of a pregnancy with multiples. Another reason for a flat head can be congenital torticollis, a condition where one of the neck muscles could be spastic and shorter on one side as a result of the *in utero* position. In this scenario, the baby tends to keep the ear bent toward the shoulder and the chin moving to the side opposite to the affected muscle, sort of tilted to the side.

Your pediatrician will help you diagnose the condition and decide if further evaluation is needed. In most cases: positional exercises, tummy time with music, sound, and color stimulation, and physical therapy with passive and active gentle stretches of the neck muscles will be enough to change the head's shape.

In severe cases, a protective custom-made helmet is applied for 20 hours a day to prevent the flattening from getting worse and even reverse it.

Please be aware, you should not attempt to experiment with turning your baby on its side while your child is asleep to avoid the flattening of the head or keep the baby on its belly in a prone position. Never put your baby at risk for SIDS.

Do not confuse the skull asymmetries of your newborn with the soft bulge over the scalp that your baby may have right after birth due to traumatic vaginal delivery, or forceps/vacuum-assisted delivery. Your pediatrician will decide what is causing the bulge, either cephalohematoma, which does not cross the suture lines and may last up to a few months, leaving a tender bump due to calcifications, or caput succedaneum, which overlaps the suture lines and is due to fluid collection that resolves within 1–2 days after birth.

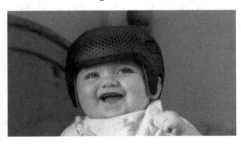

Baby with a Flat Head with Helmet

9. What should I know about breastfeeding? What foods should I avoid during lactation? What is its relationship with depression?

The period of breastfeeding can be a delightful bonding experience for most mothers, but it is also time-consuming and can lead to exhaustion, sleep deprivation, and even depression. I always encourage the family to plan on role distribution and sharing, taking turns with feedings, and if necessary, alternating latching with pumping or formula feedings depending on the health of the mother.

I will never forget when I started breastfeeding my firstborn child, my daughter Stefani, and the "let-down reflex" kicked in, the milk started to flow, but my baby was not taking to the nipples well. And in a few days, I ended up with severe mastitis (a condition caused by blocked milk ducts and bacteria entering the breast) which required treatment with oral antibiotics.

Raising a child in the late 1990s in Bulgaria was challenging. We had no electric breast pumps. After weeks of painful and resistant bacterial mastitis, hand-pumping, and applying warm compresses, I had postpartum depression and gave up on breastfeeding. I did not want to see my baby for 3 weeks, and luckily my mother was there for her and also helped me overcome my sadness. There was no awareness of postpartum depression in the '90s, and young mothers had no voice. We had to take it all in and suffer in silence. Today, I make sure all my new moms are screened for postpartum depression. There should be no shame or guilt in it, and help is available.

With my second child, my son Daniel, I used a breast pump and had milk in abundance, so much so that I had to freeze some for later use. I will never forget the day NYC had the historical blackout with no electricity for more than 48 hours due to extreme heat. I was terrified by the fact that my frozen breast milk could get spoiled and in an act of despair, loaded two duffle bags and ran into the nearest deli where the owner was using a generator. He was a young and delightful man of

Indian descent who let me take the space of the ice cream freezer and keep my breast milk there until the electricity came back on.

Every mother wants the best for their child. Lactating moms should continue their prenatal vitamins and allow for a well-balanced and nutritious diet. New parents often skip meals because of their busy schedules, but data does not show that the mother's caloric restrictions affect the quality of the breast milk. HIV medications are not recommended for use with breastfeeding. Alcohol usage needs to be tempered while breastfeeding, (e.g., after one drink of alcohol, the lactating mother should postpone breastfeeding their baby for at least 2 hours). One or 2 cups of coffee do not seem to be harmful to the baby, even though some are more sensitive and may develop intensified colic and gas.

Fish and shellfish that contain mercury must be avoided or eaten in moderation. Eight to 12 ounces of fish per week is what I recommend to my mothers, and this is supported by the American Association of Pediatricians (AAP). The quality of the fats and PUFA (polyunsaturated fatty acids or omega-3 fats) in salmon make it very valuable for the brain and eye development of the newborn. However, try to avoid tuna, swordfish, king mackerel, marlin, orange roughy, shark, and tilefish. Investigate any fish caught locally by family and friends, as well as the lake or river they were caught in, to determine if they will be safe to eat.

10. Why should I not co-sleep with my baby?

I begin to educate parents on sudden infant death syndrome (SIDS) at the baby's first newborn visit. SIDS is a common cause of unexplained death in the first months of life. Some risk factors have been studied and published, like smoking and drug use during pregnancy, lack of prenatal care, second-hand smoke exposure after birth, premature birth or extremely low birth weight, prone (belly) sleep position, soft mattresses, co-sleeping, and overheating.

Swaddling your baby after the first month poses a high risk too, perhaps because they are strong enough to roll over and get stuck in a prone position (on their bellies) which can lead to fatal suffocation.

The mattress should be as hard as possible, and no blankets, toys, or pillows should be used in the crib. Even soft crib bumpers have been associated with SIDS. Pacifiers, on the other hand, have been shown in science-based studies to be connected with the prevention of SIDS. Co-sleeping is well accepted in many cultures around the world, but especially in the first 3 months of life, the soft bedding and sheets, as well as the crowded bed could lead to accidental suffocation.

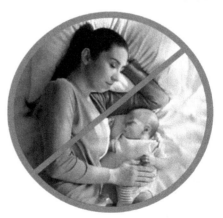

Co-sleeping

11. Why was my newborn born with a tooth, and what should I do?

I could only imagine the reaction of the parents who get to see their newborn babies for the first time and... SURPRISE, their baby has a tooth! It is quite rare as it is only seen in 1 in 2,000 births, but it happens. It is often hereditary, and chances increase if the older siblings were born with a tooth, called a natal tooth.

Malnourishment during pregnancy has been associated with increased risk, causing an impairment of the formation of dentin whose primary

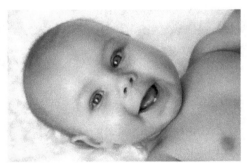

Baby with Tooth

function is to support the enamel. If the tooth is not loose and does not create difficulties with latching, there is no need to remove it. If it is loose and puts the baby at risk for choking, it will be removed by an oral surgeon. Your pediatrician will decide the next steps.

The bad news is that your nipples may get bit until they are bleeding, but the good news is you will have a smiling newborn with a precious sparkling tooth! And the latter makes for adorable pictures!

12. How should I deal with my baby's acne?

Skin lesions, including acne, are common in the newborn period. This is the time when parents are excited and obsessed with taking photos of their babies, so they are often concerned about every little bump.

Acne is not a common skin condition that I see in the first year of life. It is due to immaturity of the adrenal glands and excess production of androgen "male" hormones in the baby and partially from the androgen hormones transmitted from mom during pregnancy. It is a benign condition that should pass quickly, and unless there is a risk of scarring, I prefer the wait-and-watch approach.

Other skin conditions, especially on the face are milia, miliaria rubra, crystallina, and profunda (which are all fancy names for collections of keratin or skin flakes in the sebaceous and subcutaneous skin glands). With proper skin care and hygiene, daily baths, avoiding overheating, and using clean hypoallergenic baby products, these all conditions that resolve with time. Reassurance and compliance with the well child visits are all you need. There is nothing better than a healthy relationship with your pediatrician, based on trust and respect.

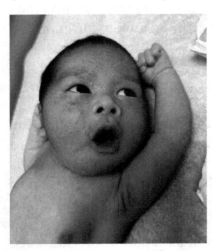

Dr. Daniela's Patient with Acne and Seborrheic Dermatitis

13. Why is my baby girl bleeding from her vagina?

It may be a scary moment when you discover that your baby girl's vagina is bleeding, until it is discussed and explained. It is known as "estrogen withdrawal syndrome," which happens when there is too much estrogen transmitted to the bloodstream of your baby girl during pregnancy. This is something that should quickly pass.

Parents are grateful when they have been warned about it in advance. The same pathophysiological mechanism stands behind the engorgement of the breasts in a newborn called "gynecomastia," which can occur in both girls and boys. Parents need to be aware that this is part of normal physiological changes and is temporary.

14. Why is my baby crying so much? How can I help them?

Believe it or not, crying loudly is normal in the first month of life, and healthy crying for up to 3 hours a day is acceptable for the first few months.

What is "healthy crying"? A strong, low-pitch cry is in fact healthy. High-pitched crying or a weak cry could be a sign of some underlying problem.

Babies cry when they are hungry, wet, or left alone because it is the only way they can communicate with their parents in the first weeks of life. Some of my parents are afraid to leave their newborn crying for a second and keep calling for consultations because they feel helpless, desperate, and sleep deprived.

Be assured that crying for up to 3 hours is more or less part of the normal development of your newborn. Of course, crying could be a sign of discomfort and a "cry for help" if your baby is hungry, colicky, has a dirty diaper, or is on the verge of a viral illness.

Some babies seem to need constant soothing and bonding with the caretaker. We are all programmed differently. Newborns are no exception, so parents have to allow time to get to know their baby patiently and lovingly. The instincts of your child are strong and you must trust them while being present for them.

15. What formula should I give to my baby?

Breast milk is your best choice for nourishment, and I encourage my parents to breastfeed until 2 years of age if they are willing to, or at the minimum for the first 6 months of life. Cow milk-based formulas are all similar and made to mimic the nutritious values of breast milk. I am not a fan of switching from cow milk based to pre-hydrolyzed hypoallergenic formulas.

If it is absolutely necessary and in cases of moderate to severe cow milk protein intolerance or allergies, your baby may require hypoallergenic formula, amino acid-based formula (in certain rare metabolic diseases), or fortified soy milk-based formula. Soy-based formula has less calcium and phosphorus, and would not be a healthy choice for at least the first 6 months of life.

All exclusively breastfed children will be prescribed 400 units of vitamin D3. Once they reach 30 ounces of formula in 24 hours the vitamin D3 drops could be discontinued. Vitamin D 3 is essential for calcium absorption and bone mineralization. Nutritional rickets leads to soft and weak bones due to insufficient calcium and vitamin D3 in the diet and is still common in developing countries.

Preterm babies have to follow the instructions of their pediatricians and stick to formula for premature babies because the ingredients and concentrations differ to provide higher caloric intake for the growing preterm. Electrolyte balance is delicate, but building the microbiome of the gut in the first three years of life is crucial for the health of your child. This starts from the first day after delivery, if not before the baby is even born.

16.Why does my baby have crossed eyes? Can my newborn see me?

"Pseudostrabismus" is the medical term for when your baby's eyes appear to be crossed. With this condition, the eyes look misaligned or crossed, but in reality, they are not. It is an illusion caused by the wider nasal bridge in babies. It is usually more noticeable and visible till 15–19 months of age. It is normal for parents to be concerned if eyes appear crossed, as strabismus (actual crossed eyes) can happen, in which case, one eye will be looking forward and the other inward or outward.

It is crucial for the pediatrician to diagnose strabismus as early as possible and make an appropriate ophthalmology referral. I like to reassure my parents and give them a quick tip on how to look at the red reflexes (when the flash of a camera lights up the blood vessels of the retina) of their children. In a photo taken while the child is looking forward, both red reflexes must be symmetrical in the center of the pupil. If they are misaligned, I advise them to bring it to my attention.

Personally, I examine the red reflexes (to identify potentially blinding but treatable disorders) of my patients on every routine visit until they are 2 years of age. The second most common reason for your baby's crossed eyes is the physiological strabismus due to immaturity of the brain and extraocular muscles, which causes transient strabismus which is outgrown around 6 months of age. If it still persists after 6 months, please talk to your doctor.

Every new parent would like to know if their newborn can see them. At birth, your newborn will have a vision of 20/200 to 20/400 (which by definition in adult patients is "legally blind"), the vision is blurry, and they can only focus in distance. They may only open their eyes in low light because of increased sensitivity to bright light. Your baby will be able to focus imperfectly on objects placed around 3-4 feet away and see across the room right after birth.

Their vision is expected to be blurry with limited focus because the eyes are still not working well together. The primary object they will be focusing on will be the parent's face at approximately 4-5 feet away from them. As they grow and their eye-hand coordination begins to develop, the infant will be tracking objects easier and looking at them, reaching out to them.

At birth, your newborn will be able to see the contrast between black and white, and after the first month, they will be able to recognize the colors red, green, orange, and yellow. If you have noticed, most toys for infants ages 0–6 months are in these shades.

17. How can I help my constipated baby? Why is my baby's diaper orange? Why does my baby have green poop? Why is my baby pooping blood?

There is nothing better than breastmilk for your newborn baby—it's that simple. Baby formulas, on the other hand, are a topic which deserves a separate book, but I will try to simplify it and make it easier to understand.

Your baby may poop after every single feeding or latching in the first 2 months, and this is not "diarrhea." Some babies poop once every 5 days, but the texture of their poop is soft and well-formed and this is not constipation. We have a variety of "normal poops" that your pediatrician will discuss with you. You may see undigested particles in the poop (seedy poop), and this is OK. Your baby is still immature and the gut needs time to develop. The pancreatic digestive enzymes are not sufficient enough for the digestion of the macronutrients (fats, protein, and carbs). Any color of poop other than white and black is normal. If your baby keeps the poop longer in the system, it may turn greener, because of the complicated process of fermentation and digestion taking place in the gastrointestinal digestive system.

Red flags for parents to watch out for include: bloody stools, white and black stools, vomiting, and decreased appetite. Some bloody and mucous-filled streaks are a sign of cow-milk protein allergy and a warning that your baby can't digest it properly. This causes inflammation of the intestines, which results in mucus and blood production.

Don't rush to switch to hypoallergenic formulas! Be aware that most of them contain corn syrup, and this may harm your baby in the long term. Evidence-based science shows around 10% increased chances of obesity later in life for children fed with formulas containing corn syrup.

Orange crystals in the diaper area are not related to bilirubin or cow milk protein allergies. They could be a sign of dehydration but are also seen in babies who are properly fed and thriving. The brick red-orangey color of the diaper is a result of urate crystals in the urine of your baby.

Nevertheless, I recommend that you call your pediatrician and ask their opinion, because you want to make sure your baby is gaining weight. Babies are rarely constipated, so please do not self-medicate with laxative suppositories as you may cause their intestines to twist and result in intestinal obstruction, which is a medical emergency. If needed, this will be done under the supervision of your pediatrician or in the ER.

18. When should I start tummy time?

When the baby is a month old, it is recommended that you begin "tummy time"—placing them on their belly so they can start lifting their head and building strength in their neck and shoulders. During the first month, you will be dealing with the umbilical stump and its care, learning how to properly burp your baby, and handling the first colicky pains. The risk for choking, along with the lack of neck and shoulder muscle strength, is a good reason to postpone tummy time till after the first month.

You can start with 2–4 minutes up to 3–5 times daily during the time your baby is awake. Right before naptime or a few minutes after you feed your baby would give them some time for proper digestion and minimize the risk of choking.

If you lay on your back and place the baby on your belly for tummy time, you can bond with your baby. You can also place musical and colorful toys in a circle to stimulate their use of neck and shoulder muscles as they look around, which will help them later on with sitting, rolling over, and crawling. Visual stimulation is another benefit of the tummy position because your baby will be able to view the world at an eye

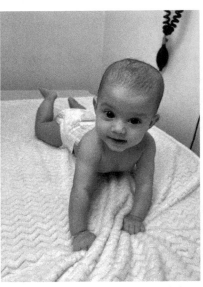

Tummy Time in Dr. Daniela's Office

level. Once tummy time becomes a part of your baby's routine you will enjoy it even more.

19. Why are my baby's legs so curved?

One of the most common questions I get from parents during their child's first year of life is, "Why are my baby's lower legs curved?" This condition is called "tibial torsion." Similar to congenital torticollis as a result of intrauterine position, one of the lower leg bones (the tibia) is internally rotated in relation to the hip. I always reassure my parents that spontaneous resolution between 1 and 4 years of age is the most common outcome. Follow-ups and annual physical exams by the pediatrician are sufficient.

When the infant starts walking, mild in-toeing (walking with the toes turned toward the opposite foot) is noticed but there is no need for podiatry or physical therapy referrals. If the tibial torsion is asymmetrical, or there is leg length discrepancy, an appropriate referral to an orthopedic surgeon must be done. In rare cases, the curvature is due to Blount's disease, which is when the growth plate near the knee stops making new bone and the curvature is severe and progressively getting worse. Surgical evaluation and treatment are indicated.

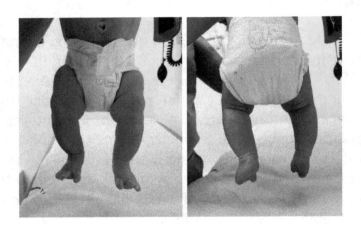

Dr. Daniela's Patient with Tibial Torsion (Front and Back View)

20. Why is my baby spitting up, crying hysterically, and hunching over?

To all moms, dads, parents, and caretakers: it is normal for your newborn baby to be spitting up and vomiting occasionally. Once your baby is delivered and the umbilical cord is cut and clamped, you will be able to bond with your baby and breastfeed them in about one hour after delivery. Latching is an instinct for survival and comes easily, but for some babies born prematurely or with significant genetic, metabolic disorders, or anatomic defects, latching, and feeding could present a challenge. Most hospitals provide latching counseling right after birth.

At the first visit, I always educate my parents that spitting up is a normal physiological response due to immature and weak muscles at the end of the esophagus (feeding tube). Most of the time your baby will spit up when they are burped and sometimes even vomit small amounts. Some babies latch too fast or swallow gas, while others are overfed by their parents.

As long as your baby is thriving, gaining weight, and wetting 8–10 diapers in 24 hours, I would not be alarmed.

However, if vomiting is projectile and happens after every feeding, it needs to be addressed immediately. There is a condition called "pyloric stenosis" in which the muscles of the part of the stomach that connects to the intestines are in spasm, preventing the digested food from moving down to the gut. Another common clinical scenario would be persistent vomiting, which leads to lack of weight gain also known as "failure to thrive." If your baby can't keep the milk down, is not gaining weight, and is constantly hungry and fussy, your doctor may tell you that the baby has acid reflux (GERD or gastroesophageal reflux) that needs to be treated. My initial advice is to offer smaller but more frequent feedings to help with this, and in older babies, around 4 months of age, thickening the breast milk/formula with rice or oatmeal cereal could be an option. Do not attempt to change any feeding patterns before consulting with your pediatrician first.

21. Why are my baby's eyes tearing up?

About 6–10% of newborns tear up without crying, and parents wonder why. The nasolacrimal duct canals are the tiny little tubes or "pipes" where the tears travel after stimulation of the lacrimal glands. The canals have two valves that sometimes malfunction because of embryonic remnants, which cause the canals to obstruct and cause dacryostenosis or inflammation of the tear duct canals. Most commonly, it is a congenital condition that resolves spontaneously around 9–12 months of age.

I advise my parents to apply gentle massage over the nasolacrimal duct canals 2–3 times daily for about 2–3 minutes. Rarely, if the condition persists beyond 1 year of age, probing (procedure to open the canals) would be performed by an ophthalmologist. Infections may occur, and if there is redness of the conjunctivae (the mucous membrane that covers the front of the eye and inside the eyelids) and if it has yellowish eye discharge, you have to notify your pediatrician. If both valves are malfunctioning, a cyst can form, which looks like a reddish, tender lump in the inner corner of the eye. This condition, also diagnosed as "dacryocystocele," requires immediate medical attention. Tears are protective to the eyes and keep them lubricated and healthy, so healthy tear ducts are important.

22. Why does my baby have a stuffy nose?

Newborns have tiny nasal canals and instinctively breathe through their nostrils only, so any nasal congestion will cause them to make funny noises and struggle with latching and/or bottle feedings. As humans, we are built to breathe through our nostrils which filter and moisturize the air.

Any temperature or humidity change, dust, second-hand smoking, chemicals, and air contamination may cause a buildup of mucus and cause nasal congestion. Your newborn won't be able to breathe using their mouth in the first few months to facilitate their latching and keeping the milk down the feeding tube. Slowly, with time they do learn how to separate the tongue from the hard palate.

My best advice for parents is to use nasal saline 0.65% solution (hypotonic) in the form of drops. Use 2–3 drops in each nostril before feedings if you have noticed that your newborn is congested. You don't have to aggressively suction the nose; let the saline irrigate the sinuses and provide some relief. It's like showering your nasal canals. I recommend using saline drops (not the spray) to avoid nosebleeds as the blood vessels (the Kiesselbach plexus, in the anterior part of the nose) in the first month of life are very fragile and can break down under the pressure of nasal spray release, which can cause nosebleeds.

Some cultures practice taping the mouth or closing it to stimulate the development of proper nostril breathing. They may even tape the mouths of their children while asleep, which is dangerous as it can prevent breathing and lead to death.

23. Is it safe to introduce solids to my baby? How do I start if they don't have teeth yet?

The American Association for Pediatrics (AAP) recommends introducing solids between 4 to 6 months of age. Most babies start the teething process around 3–4 months of age. They salivate more, drool, and keep their fists in their mouths. On average, the first tooth will erupt around 6 months of age, but the ranges of normal vary. Your baby does not have to have teeth to chew food and swallow it.

Carefully prepared pureed or fork-mashed foods should be offered initially. If your baby is choking and having trouble chewing the food, you may hold off a bit and try again another time. In premature babies or kids with neurodevelopmental delays, solid food readiness might be delayed.

The "extrusion reflex" does not last beyond 5 months. This is the innate reflex that involves raising the tongue to push out food and anything else that is placed in the child's mouth. Persistence of the extrusion reflex makes spoon feeding frustrating for both the parents and the infant.

24.   When should I introduce water to my baby? How much should I give them?

Breast milk is about 87% water, so if your baby is exclusively breastfed, the recommended age for water introduction is 6 months. The nutrients in breastmilk and formula are all that your baby needs, and adding water too soon may lead to electrolyte imbalances and hyponatremia (below normal blood sodium level) which could possibly cause brain damage.

Your baby's electrolyte balance is very delicate, and an imbalance can compromise the function of major organs like the brain, kidneys, and liver. Parents must pay close attention to the instructions on how to dilute baby formula.

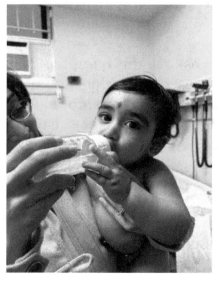
Baby Getting Water in a Bottle in Dr. Daniela's Office

With the introduction of solids around 6 months, breastfed and formula-fed babies are offered water initially in small amounts 4-8 ounces daily, and this can be gradually increased.

Tap water could be contaminated or

contain lead, and boiling it just increases the concentration of lead in the water because some of the water will evaporate. Using filtered, deionized, demineralized, distilled, or bottled water is your best choice. In developing countries, boiling water is part of culture, but contaminated water use is never alright.

25. When can my baby start sitting in a high chair?

My patients like to ask me this question. They worry about the baby's back, breathing, and head control. Most high chairs have been approved for 6 months of age and older, and they have a maximum weight listed.

As soon as your baby has stable head control without head lag (which is a milestone they reach at 4–5 months) and is able to sit with support or independently, they can be safely placed in a high chair. This is also the time we start introducing solids. If your baby is comfortably sitting in the chair, can accept a spoonful of pureed food, and swallows without choking, you can start using the high chair. Their hands should be freely moving so you can allow them to explore and stimulate the development of their fine motor skills, like self-feeding, opening their mouth, and chewing.

The back of the seat must not be reclined. You may feel that moving the seat backwards would provide more stability for the head, but it may obstruct the airways. Your baby is still developing their gross motor skills. Occupational therapists like to use the 90-90-90 rule, meaning that the hips, knees, and feet should all be positioned at a 90-degree angle. The feet of your baby must not be hanging in the air but rather have nice support for improved stability.

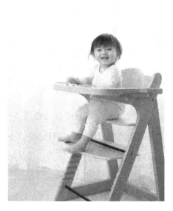
Toddler in a Highchair

NOTE: These are happy and messy times. Don't forget to document with video and photographs all precious moments!

26. What should I do about "cradle cap"? Does my baby have oral thrush if their tongue is white?

The medical term for "cradle cap" is "seborrhea capitis." It can be easily confused with eczema or atopic dermatitis. In the first month of their lives, 10% of newborns have this condition. It usually resolves by 4 to 6 weeks but can be observed until the 1st year of life.

Cradle cap looks like small yellowish-silver plaques that start accumulating in the scalp hair area, behind the ears, neck and eyebrows. Occasionally, the lesions can spread to the trunk, arms, and back areas and can even be seen in the mouth as oral thrush or in the diaper area as diaper rash. There are a few reasons for the accumulation of these scaly plaques. The androgens ("male" hormones) transmitted to the newborn during pregnancy stimulate the sebaceous glands that lead to the increased production of sebum, the oily substance your skin makes that keeps it from drying out.

An overgrowth of *Malassezia*, a type of fungus that thrives in a greasy (lipid) environment has been blamed for these conditions as well. For more severe cases of cradle cap, with an inflammatory element, I usually prescribe Ketoconazole 2% or Selsun Blue 3% shampoo or lotion, which are both antifungal topical options. Your pediatrician will walk you through the exact process of application. Topical steroids may be needed, but your doctor will ultimately be the decision maker.

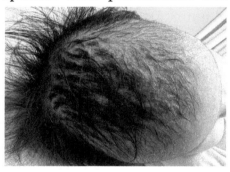

Baby with Cradle Cap

For the most part, cradle cap is an asymptomatic and self-resolving condition that requires only application of baby oils such as Aquaphor (Petrolatum) for 5 minutes prior to bathtime and overnight. A gentle brushing of the scalp with a soft hair or tooth brush helps remove the accumulated plaques.

Although parents tend to be the first to notice oral thrush, it is not unusual for the condition to be mistaken for milk accumulation that appears as a thick white plaque on the tongue's surface. *Candida albicans* accumulates in the oral flora and could be transmitted from the skin of mom's nipples during latching or from contaminated pacifiers, bottles, and even the dropper of the vitamin D3 bottles. Your doctor will decide if

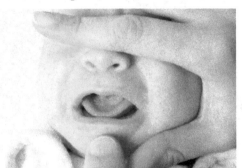

Baby with Oral Thrush

treatment is needed, but as soon as you notice white plaques of the tongue and/or the buccal mucosa (the inside of the cheeks) and

the posterior phalanx (the back of the throat) call your pediatrician. If left untreated, the fungus can spread down to the esophagus (the digestive feeding tube) and cause maldigestion, vomiting, and esophagitis (inflammation of the esophagus). Liquid antifungal medications are easily available for the latter diagnosis and will be prescribed by your pediatrician if needed.

27. When should I start the "cry it out" method?

The "cry it out" (CIO) method has been studied for many decades and there are different methods described in the literature: Weissbluth, Murkoff, Ezzo and Bucknam, Hogg and Blau, Ferber, Giordano, and Abirdin are among the experts in this method. What differs is the approach and the starting age of the training technique. Regardless of what method you or your pediatrician chooses, there are a few simple rules you have to stick to when sleep training.

If there is more than one parent (caretaker) in the home, before you are ready for the CIO trial, everyone must be on the same page to avoid conflicts between themselves and confusion for the baby's immature brain. Once the parent(s) commit to it, you have to begin the process and follow it till your baby fully adopts the new way of self-soothing and falling asleep. Your baby has very short sleep cycles, lasting 50–60 minutes, and every time they wake up, will expect the same soothing rituals they are used to (rocking, cuddling, feeding) to go back to sleep. CIO is controversial, but most pediatricians agree that your baby is developmentally ready to start the training between 4–6 months. Once you are assured that your baby is well-fed, healthy, and gaining weight, you can start initiating bedtime routines with a warm bath, massage, soothing music, and a story. You can gently place the child in the crib and leave them alone while drowsy and not fully asleep. Gradually increasing the amount of time that you let them cry will slowly teach them how to independently go back to sleep.

The CIO method does not mean that you have to abandon your baby. You should start the process slowly (start with 1–2 minutes), gradually increasing the amount of time before you check on your child. You can pick them up for a moment and place them back in the crib while they are still awake. The goal is to develop new associations in your baby's brain during this transitional stage so they can learn how to go back to sleep on their own. Proponents of this method argue that it can lead to better sleep habits for both the baby and parents, while opponents raise concerns about potential negative effects on the emotional baby's well-being.

Every baby is different, and what works for one family may not work for another. Proceed with caution, listening to your baby's needs and sensitivity. You can always interrupt the training and get back to it in a few weeks or months if it becomes overwhelming and emotionally draining to the family (Bilgen & Wolke, 2020).

28. How do I know if my newborn is well-fed?

This is a question I get on every first visit when I get to meet a newborn. Your baby will be guiding you in the first months. Their physiological needs will be met if you offer your breast on demand, considering you produce sufficient amounts of milk. How do you know if it is sufficient?

Offering each breast for 15–20 minutes during a single feeding, or pumping and feeding your baby by a bottle with either formula or breast milk is done on demand in the first 3-6 weeks of life. A simple rule is offering approximately 2 ounces every 2 hours, 3 ounces every 3 hours, 4 ounces every 4 hours. (One ounce equals 28 ml, but you can approximate this to 30 ml to simplify the math.)

Another way to find out if your baby is sufficiently fed is by measuring the wet diapers–if you go through 7–12 wet diapers in 24 hours, this indicates that your baby is getting enough food.

In the first months of life, your newborn will be weighed every 2-4 weeks in the pediatrician's office. Your baby will leave the nursery a bit lighter compared to their birth weight but will quickly regain it around 10–14 days. Your newborn will likely experience a growth spurt in the first 3 months; this is more prominent in breastfed babies compared to formula-fed babies. Your baby should double their weight by around 5 months of age and triple it by 1 year.

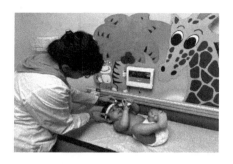

Measuring Baby's Head in Dr. Daniela's Office

29. Can I offer my breastfed baby a pacifier?

"Nipple confusion" or "nipple preference" are terms used to describe the fussiness some babies exhibit when switched form the breast to the bottle nipple, which some parents may be concerned about for breastfed babies who may need a pacifier.

According to La Leche League, there is no way to predict who will have problems breastfeeding after drinking from a bottle or using a pacifier. You may wait until breastfeeding is well established to let them try a pacifier. Using a pacifier is soothing, though, and (believe it or not) it has been shown in some research studies to be protective against SIDS (Moon et al., 2012).

Your baby needs milk. By offering a pacifier you are not interfering with their instinct to latch and feed. A healthy newborn will be able to take the breast unless the mother has inverted nipples or clogged milk ducts or if the baby is tongue-tied (can't move their tongue well due to a short

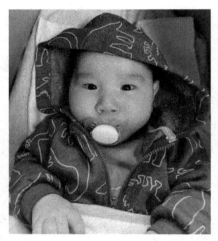

Dr. Daniela's Patient with a Pacifier

band of tissue that connects the tongue to the mouth) or has genetic facial defects like cleft lip/palate or other neurodevelopmental and metabolic diseases. I do encourage moms to seek the expertise of latching specialists if needed. Breastfeeding is simply natural, but it's not always easy and this is why you have the support of your pediatrician and lactation consultant.

30. How do I burp my child? What should I do for a colicky or fussy baby?

Burping after every feeding, regardless of whether it's with a breast or bottle, is essential for the wellbeing of your baby. Your newborn is in the process of learning how to latch/drink without swallowing too much gas. Building up gas in the stomach and the intestines will lead to colic and fussiness. Lactating mothers may notice their nipples sore, cracked, and bleeding, and if your newborn happens to swallow some blood,

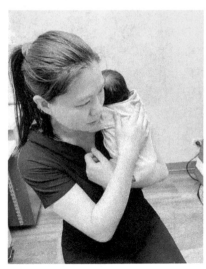

Performing Burping Technique
(On the Mother's Shoulder)

it won't harm them.

The latching specialists in the hospital will review all burping techniques and proper ways of holding your baby during feedings, holding the bottle properly, and choosing the right bottle. Gently tapping the baby's back while holding them on your shoulder in an upright position or holding them on your lap, bending forward from sitting position by supporting the chin, are the most commonly used methods and are recommended by the AAP.

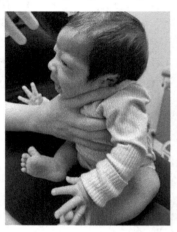

Performing Burping Technique (Front Facing with Chin Support and Bending Forward)

As I have reviewed earlier in this chapter, "colic" is a normal physiological process and requires time and patience. Every baby is different, and you need not compare. With the support of your partner and caretaker and the professional advice of your pediatrician, you will be able to overcome the stressful period of your colicky and fussy baby.

31. Should I circumcise my son? Why is my child's penis not growing? Why are there white bumps on my son's penis?

I leave the choice of circumcision to the parents and their cultural and religious beliefs. I do provide them with the latest research and the AAP recommendations. There is proof that circumcision is beneficial in preventing penis cancer, STDs, and in rare occasions, urinary tract infections. Following good hygiene is enough to help prevent all of the above-mentioned diseases, though.

At the same time, teaching your boy how to properly clean his private parts, immunizing with human papillomavirus (HPV) vaccines, and using protection during sexual intercourse later on in life, would be enough to keep them disease-free.

I work in one of the most culturally diverse areas in the world (which is Elmhurst and Jackson

Heights, Queens, New York) where approximately 180,000 residents speak over 160 languages. Because of my work setting, I have developed a strong sense of respect toward all cultures and religious rituals. I always tell my parents that they are the ultimate decision-makers, and I am there to support and help them.

If your baby's penis is not growing or is not visible, there could actually be excess fat accumulation in the pubic area or in chubbier kids later in life.

Occasionally my parents will come after noticing white bumps on the baby's penis. These are dead epithelial skin cells trapped under the foreskin, called "preputial cysts." It's a totally benign condition. With time, once the foreskin is fully retracted, the cystic lesions will be pushed out. There is no special care needed, and manipulation or removing of the cysts is not advisable, because it could be harmful for the child.

32. Why does my baby have a red spot on the back of the scalp? What is a "café au lait" spot?

Is the birthmark of your baby a "kiss from an angel"? Many cultures believe that their baby was blessed by God or an angel and is special when born with a birthmark. There are so many different interpretations of matching birthmarks to personality traits. In fact, birthmarks occur randomly, and in limited cases can lead to a more serious diagnosis.

The common "salmon patch" mostly observed over the middle of the forehead or the back of the neck is simply an area with superficial capillaries that fade with time.

The "Mongolian blue spots" described first in the Asian and Mongolian populations (with the belief that they are more common among the Asian race) can also be seen in any race and they also slowly fade with time.

Hemangiomas are larger and elevated, involving blood vessel dilation, and if they cover sensitive areas like the eyes, nose, mouth, or private areas, require treatment.

Café au lait spots are brownish random marks with no clinical significance except if they are multiple and part of a common genetic disease called neurofibromatosis.

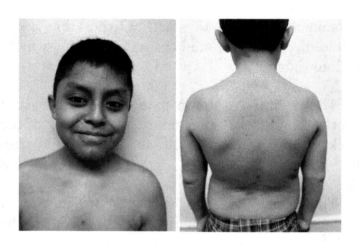

Neurofibromatosis-Type 1 *Cafe au Lait* Spots on the Face and Trunk (From the Front and Back)

Hypopigmented patches also could be insignificant or part of tuberous sclerosis.

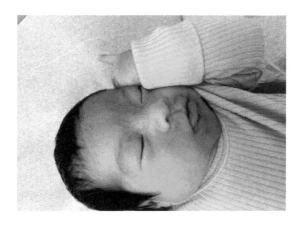

Baby with Left Nostril and Forehead Hemangiomas

Melanocytes are the cells responsible for melanin which gives the color of the birthmark and our skin. Regardless of the origin of the birthmark, there is either a vascular or concentration of melanocytes presented as hyperpigmentations or there is a lack of melanocytes presented as hypopigmentations. Your pediatrician will decide if your child needs further evaluation and intervention.

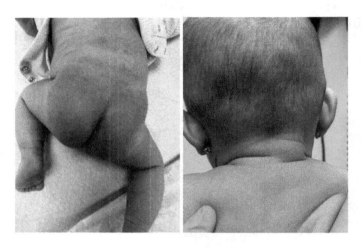

Baby's Back with a
Mongolian Spot

Baby's Neck with a
Hemangioma or "Salmon
Patch"

33.   When can I pierce my baby's ears?

Ear piercing is a very common practice among cultures throughout the world; however, significant disparities exist about when to pierce the ears and how often families involve their pediatricians in making this decision. When families do choose to involve their provider, there are some important elements to discuss with them about the timing and possible complications of ear piercing.

The timing of ear piercing can often be influenced by a family's culture or traditions. The American Academy of Pediatrics most recent writing on this topic dates back to 2004 and notes, "[...] as a general guideline, postpone the piercing until your child is mature enough to take care of the pierced site herself." Like many parenting and medical decisions, the question of timing is one of risk versus benefit. The AAP further advises, "[...] if the piercing is performed carefully and cared for conscientiously, there is little risk."

Clean the ear piercing area with alcohol, and use topical anesthetic if possible, then accurately measure the earring placement before the sterile piercing needle device is used. Ensure that the earrings are not too tight to avoid redness and inflammation, or even more serious complications like cellulitis that should be treated with antibiotics.

The material of the earrings is important. Sterling silver and gold are ideal if you want to avoid contact dermatitis caused by nickel-based materials. Keeping the pierced ears clean and dry and applying topical antibiotics sometimes prescribed by your pediatrician will prevent infection. Using a non-medical gun device in places other than the pediatric office can cause tissue trauma and keloid formation. Parents should change to permanent earrings in 4-6 weeks to assure the healing is complete.

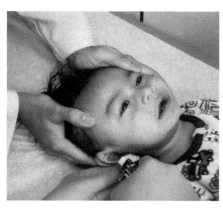

A Toddler Getting her Ears Pierced in Dr. Daniela's Office using Sterile Needle Medical Device

Even though in some countries the newborn can leave the hospital with their ears pierced, my recommendation is to wait at least until 4 months, after the first series of Hepatitis B and DtaP have been administered.

Performing the procedure in a sterile environment like the doctor's office is advisable.

34. Why do my baby's nipples have white milk-like discharge? Why does my baby have an extra nipple?

Most newborns will have mild tenderness and engorgement of the breasts as discussed earlier in the book. When parents touch the breasts and nipples, they often panic because they feel that, "something is growing under the nipples." This is not a mass; this is part of the mammary gland that is enlarged due to the elevated estrogen levels transmitted during the pregnancy from mom.

Thin milk-like fluid could also be expressed from the breasts, called "galactorrhea" for the same reasons or in medical terminology known as "estrogen withdrawal syndrome." It is common both in girls and boys, could be asymmetric, and resolves with time around 4-6 weeks of age.

Extra nipples or "supernumerary nipples" are not as rare as you may think. I have trained my eyes during my career to spot those small rudimentary (inactive) nipples or nipples with underlying breast tissue that look like a birthmark, but if you feel them gently, they appear to have a small dimple that differs from a birthmark. The most common location is above or below the breasts, along the nipple line. There is no need for concern, and they will just look like a small birthmark and never become an actual "nipple."

Sometimes nipples and breasts can be spaced out too wide. In this case, the pediatrician may conduct a genetic test to rule out Turner syndrome if they have concerns about the nipples. Turner syndrome is a condition that affects only females and results when one of the sex chromosomes (X chromosomes) is partially or fully missing. Turner syndrome only affects 3% of all female babies.

35. Should I give my baby Tylenol just before and/or after a vaccination appointment?

In some countries around the world, it is still a common practice to medicate the baby before administering vaccines. Lots of evidence-based studies have been published against using Tylenol (acetaminophen) during or within the first 4 hours after vaccination and these are the current guidelines of AAP and the World Health Organization.

Unless your baby reacts to the vaccines and develops a fever higher than 101°F or 38.5°C, or is extremely fussy and inconsolable, there is no need to administer fever control medications, even after vaccinating, because you don't want to interfere with the immune system and interrupt the production of sufficient antibodies for future prevention.

Local reactions are common, and all they need is a cool compress within 24 hours of the inoculation. If the redness observed around the injection site is as large as an egg, tender, and warm when you touch it, contact your pediatrician immediately.

Every country has different vaccine calendars and recommendations. If you plan to travel with your children, consult with your doctor a few months prior to find out what vaccines are needed and allow time for immunity to build up.

36.   When do I introduce them to solids?

The American Academy of Pediatrics (AAP) recommends that you start introducing solids between 4 and 6 months of age. It is a lengthy process and you have to allow 1 to 2 days for every new food you introduce. There is no specific order you need to follow, but I advise my parents to start with the basic groups of fruits and vegetables, one at a time for 2 days in a row and if there are no allergic reactions (vomiting, skin rashes, and/or diarrhea), you can move on to the next food.

Once you let your child experience the taste and texture of the fruits and veggies, you can add meats, fish, seafood, shellfish, eggs, peanut butter, and baby yogurt.

There is no right or wrong food with the exception to avoid honey and regular cow milk until after 1 year of age. Honey must be avoided because of the risk of botulism, a toxic bacteria that grows in the honey and could be lethal to your baby. Regular cow milk can lead to iron deficiency anemia because the calcium in the milk competes with iron absorption in the gut.

The goal is to expand the palate of your baby, develop a healthy microbiome and reduce the chances of future allergic reactions by introducing your baby to as many common food allergens as possible at an early age.

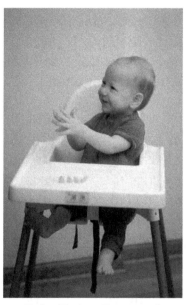

Your baby will be able to take a teaspoon and digest pureed food, but you must be careful to avoid choking by feeding with big chunks

Baby Eating Quartered Grapes

of food, offering whole peanuts, grapes, cherries, etc.

Juice is not recommended in the first year of life, even though in many cultures around the globe, juice is the first food other than milk offered around the age of 4 months. If your child is sneezing, coughing, choking, or gagging after feedings, please consult your pediatrician immediately. I personally witnessed a case of sneezing 10 to 15 minutes after feedings because of a missed cleft palate.

Offer the solids before the milk bottle feedings or before you offer the breast for a particular meal. This will allow your baby to enjoy the solids and explore the textures and tastes. Feeding difficulties are not uncommon, but should be discussed with your pediatrician as they could be a sign of a medical condition, or could indicate behavioral and/or developmental problems or illnesses—for instance, children on the autism spectrum often present with difficulties with feeding.

CHAPTER TWO: DEVELOPMENT AND GROWTH

Dr. Shellie's Mom Memories of Child Development and Growth

Both of my children grew physically very well and were at a healthy height and weight from the beginning. But their social and emotional growth, and willingness to challenge themselves intellectually, were different between the two of them from the start.

Alyssa was hitting her developmental milestones in record time. At the daycare when she was 4 years old they had to grab puzzles from the 1st grade room because she could always see things a few steps ahead and needed the intellectual stimulation.

Jacob, on the other hand, struggled with some of the social-emotional benchmarks, and we could see at an early age that he needed much more guidance and saw the world through a different lens. He interacted with other children through "parallel play" instead of playing directly with them. He would mostly play beside them, and there were often misunderstandings due to Jacob missing social cues.

There was a point in my career when I was a tenured education professor at a private university where I was considered to be an expert on children with special needs. When Jacob was diagnosed with ADHD, I was not surprised at all. However, it took a talk with a relative who had raised a child on the autism spectrum, wherein they compared Jacob's quirky ways with their own child that I decided to get him tested for autism spectrum disorder (ASD). I have always suggested to students (when I was a professor of future teachers) and parents (when I was a teacher and when I was an assistant principal of children with emotional and behavioral needs) that, if you suspect that the child needs extra support due to a special need, you need to get them tested early through your pediatrician's *recommendation because early intervention services are profoundly helpful for the child's coping skills and setting them on the right track for success. But even as a so-called "expert," I feel I slightly delayed the testing because I had been naturally and instinctively making accommodations for his needs, and his future diagnosis was not really obvious to me during the first five years of his life.*

Make sure you give yourself grace with these types of parenting issues. Realize that all children learn and develop at different paces. They have their own personalities and rates of growth. If you are given a diagnosis by a medical professional, make sure that you either write it down, record it on your phone, or bring a trusted friend with you so you can recall the information, instructions, and suggestions later. You are going to support your child and help the professionals who will work with them differentiate to meet their individualized needs!

Dr. Daniela's Pediatric Prescription for Child Development and Growth

37. Why is my child not cooing or babbling?

Cooing or making vowel sounds and vocalizing upon hearing others are the first signs of communication, perhaps second only to crying that you will observe and hear. At 1 month of age, your baby should be able to react to sounds. You will see their reactions when they turn their heads and startle at loud noises like slamming the door or loud music or speech. Cooing is a milestone that babies develop and master around 2 months of age. At 3–4 months, your baby will be turning toward voices and laughing out loud. At 6 months you will start hearing your baby babble (making consonant vowels).

At 9 months, most babies can put two syllables together, but they are not specifically addressing "mama" and "dada." Do not take it personally, but most of the time "dada" comes first because it is much easier to use the tongue and the palate to make the "d" sound instead of using the lips for "mama." At 12 months of age, your baby should be able to address "mama" and "dada" specifically by calling them, looking at them, and recognizing them.

If you notice delays, share them with your pediatrician. I review all milestones at every visit and address any delays with speech immediately. It also could be an initial sign of autism or other developmental delays. Early intervention, close observation, banning screen time, and stimulating the brain development and speech are essential.

38. Should I be concerned if my 1-year-old is not addressing me with "mama" or their father with "dada" specifically? Should I be concerned if my child isn't speaking in full sentences by 2?

The answer to these questions is "yes," you should share your concerns with your pediatrician. Babies start to coo at the ages of 2–3 months, babble at 5–6 months, and start saying "mama," "papa," and "dada" nonspecifically at 9 months of age. When they are 1 year old, I expect my little patients to be able to address "Mama" and "Dada" specifically and at 15 to 18 months they should add 5 words in addition to "mama" and "dada."

At 2 years of age, they should be able to make simple 2-word sentences, address you, follow 2-step commands, and add 50–100 words to their vocabulary.

At 2–3 years of age, your child should be able to construct two- or three-word sentences and have a vocabulary of 200 to 500 words. Caregivers will be able to understand 50% of the speech of their 2-year-old and 75% of a 3-year-old child. At 4 years of age, 100% of the speech should be understandable by both familiar people (caregivers) and unfamiliar people (strangers).

Every child is unique and develops at their own pace, but it is up to your pediatrician to assess and evaluate. Checking the hearing is the first step, and if not offered by your provider, please ask for it. After ruling out hearing deficits, your toddler should follow up with a full developmental test (ideally provided by an EIP, early intervention program, or developmental specialist) and if there are no associated developmental delays, speech therapy must be initiated.

Limiting screen time until 2 years of age is something I recommend to all my patients. We live surrounded by electronics, and screens are everywhere. Technology overuse affects our children negatively in many aspects, inhibits their social skills, delays speech and affects relationships, causes loneliness, and plays a major role in depression among teens and young adults. Living with robots, smartphones, iPads, computers, and smartwatches can affect memory and lead to comprehension deficits and learning difficulties in school.

Parents must adjust their schedules and find time for their children. Human interaction and age appropriate brain stimulation games are what children need and would appreciate. Do not forget that they fully depend on us, the ADULTS, their parents, relatives, teachers, and doctors.

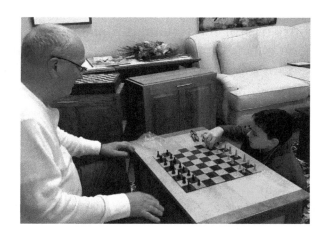

Dr. Shellie's Son and his Grandfather Playing Chess

39. Why is my toddler walking pigeon-toed (toes pointing in)? Why is my 3-year-old still tip-toeing?

There is not a day in my office that goes by without encountering a question concerning toddlers' and preschoolers' gaits and the way that they walk. Some of my parents start pointing out the inward position of the feet from the moment their children begin standing even before walking.

The feet are connected to the bones of the lower leg, consisting of the tibia and fibula, which is the shinbone. The tibia is the larger bone sitting medially or closer to the center of the body. The tibia and fibula are then connected to the knee joint and the femoral bone or thighbone. The connections are made by tendons and ligaments to hold the bones together and stabilize them.

While in the womb, the embryo is in fetal position with the tibial bones flexed internally which causes the feet to also rotate inward. Tibial torsion was discussed previously but it is closely tied to in-toeing in toddlers and children. The alignment of the bones is a smooth process that occurs naturally during the first 4–5 years of life and rarely needs intervention. Braces, casting, or orthotics are rarely recommended because this is a normal physiological process of growth and development of coordination and balance.

As long as the in-toeing is not affecting the child's movement and is not painful, it does not require any restrictions or concern. If it persists above 5 years of age; is accompanied by pain, frequent falls, or tripping; or prevents the child from playing sports, a podiatrist and orthopedic surgeon may be involved in the case.

Often, preschool teachers and relatives ask a child's parents to seek medical advice if the child is walking on their toes. In fact, children like to experiment and as soon as they begin to bear weight they may occasionally show a preference for cruising (which is the stage between crawling and walking) or walking on their toes.

By the age of 2, the heal-to-toe gait pattern is established, and if your child continues to tip-toe until after 3–5 years of age a medical consult may be advisable. Most children outgrow this habit by the age of 5, keeping in mind that extended tip-toeing may lead to stiffening of the Achilles tendon. This could be easily treated with physical therapy and stretching exercises.

It is extremely rare for a child with inward toeing or tip-toeing to be diagnosed with a neuropsychiatric or developmental disease. Reassurance and observation is the main approach to this type of common occurrence.

40. Is my baby gaining weight too fast? Why is my newborn not putting on weight?

In the first 1 to 2 hours of delivering your baby, you can start offering your breast. This is going to be your first intimate interaction with your newborn. In the first 3 months of life, your newborn will have a growth spurt, which is more noticeable in breastfed babies, compared to formula-fed. Your baby won't typically grow too fast or gain too much weight unless there is an underlying medical or genetic condition.

Every time you visit your pediatrician at the well baby visits, the growth curve of your child will be plotted and reviewed. The weight gain of your baby depends on the intrauterine environment and maternal nutrition during and after pregnancy, if breastfeeding. There are three measurements that are the most important and are followed on the growth curve: weight, height, and head circumference. If your baby is growing healthily, the measurements will follow the curve progression smoothly with only slight deviations from the curve.

Even though breastfed babies gain weight more rapidly in the first 3 months of life, the weights are similar by 12–23 months of life. The expected weight gain in the first 3 months is about an ounce per day (30 grams), from months 3-6, .7 ounces per day (20 grams), and from months 6–12 of age, .35 ounces per day (10 grams). Infants double their weight by the age of 5 to 6 months and triple it in their first year of life. After the age of 2 years, we estimate approximately 5 pounds (2.3 kg) of weight gain per year until puberty.

Every child has a different genetic growth potential. Most children grow in a predictable fashion, but if they lack growth or weight gain, it should be addressed. Poor weight gain is common, and some causes are prematurity, congenital anomalies (like cleft lip or palate or chromosomal disorders), intrauterine exposure to alcohol or drugs, exposure to lead, and iron deficiency anemia. Social isolation, mental illness, stress, poor parental skills, violence, and abuse are among some of the factors that can lead to poor weight gain.

Globally in 2020, 45 million children were estimated to be too thin for their height, and 45% of deaths among children under 5 years of age are linked to malnutrition (a deficiency of nutrients) (World Health Organization, 2021a).

41. Should I stop my son from playing with dolls and wearing his sister's dresses? How do I talk to my child about gender differences?

Young children who play with dolls often grow up to be good and caring parents. Wearing a dress will not hurt your child. Embrace your child's love for imaginative play. This type of exploration doesn't set their sexuality or gender orientation.

The evolution of medicine and science has certainly affected our perception of the body and disease. It has affected our way of living, the way we communicate, and the relationship between parents and children. The moment children discover their private parts is the moment when their sparkling curiosity is ignited. Around the age of 3, most children identify strongly with gender, including transgender and gender non-conforming children.

You may need to be prepared to answer questions like, "Am I a boy, or am I a girl?" or "Can a baby have two moms or two dads?" and it is ok to be honest with your child. At the time of press on this book, in the United States, more than 10 states allow parents to choose a gender-neutral option on their child's birth certificate. As parents, we need to leave it up to the child and their natural growth and development so they can express how they feel in their own bodies and determine their gender and pronouns later in life.

Over the centuries, genders have been stereotyped, and it was believed that there are only two genders: male and female or boy and girl. Historically in most Western cultures, blue was the color for boys, pink for girls; cars were boys' toys, and Barbies were girls' toys; pants were for boys, and skirts and dresses for girls; short hair for boys and long for girls. Boys were supposed to be the stronger gender, never cry, or show emotion in public.

Society, culture, and religions have different understanding and acceptance of the fluidity of gender identity. It is an ethical question for some and may create rejection and hatred, leading to mental health illnesses in your growing child. Be open, try to support your child's interests, and seek medical help if you have difficulties understanding your child's choices. If your child does identify as LGBTQ+ in the future, listen with a caring heart and strive to love them unconditionally.

42. Can you predict how tall your child will be as an adult?

The average height of a healthy, full-term born baby is 20 inches (50 cm). Infants grow 10 inches (25 cm) during the first year of life, and toddlers grow 4 inches (10 cm) between 12 and 24 months, 3 inches (7.5 cm) between 24 and 48 months.

Two common causes of short stature after the first 2 years of life are familial and constitutional short stature, both with a normal pace of growth.

The most common question from parents I encounter is, "How tall will my child be?" There is a formula that helps us predict the average height based on height after the 2nd year of life. Subtract 5 in (13 cm) from the father's height for females, and average it with the mother's height. For males, add 5 in (13 cm) to the mother's height, and then average that with the father's height. There are exceptions to the rule. This is an approximate formula that does not predict or include environmental factors and underlying conditions. Because growth has to do with hormones, children with delayed growth should see an endocrinologist.

43. When will my baby get their first teeth?

Teeth formation starts during the 6th week in utero and continues until adolescence. The 20 primary or "baby teeth" formation and eruption begins between 6 and 10 months of age, while the permanent 32 teeth start erupting around 6 years of age.

When teething, your baby will be fussy, put their fists in their mouth, and chew on their blanket or toys. To prevent choking hazards, we do not recommend allowing the baby to wear necklaces, anklets, or bracelets, as those will be easily reached and placed in the mouth. Chewing on a single cold teething ring will be the safest and most soothing way to help your baby through teething.

AAP does not support any of the OTC holistic remedies or topical viscous lidocaine or Orajel containing benzocaine, as they have been associated with side effects and poisoning (methemoglobinemia). Teething is a natural and physiological process of growth and development that does not need to be medicated. Your baby will learn how to cope and deal with pain.

Your fussy teething baby may experience low-grade fever, but anything above 100.4°F (38°C) must be discussed with your pediatrician. You don't want to miss a serious viral or bacterial infection by simply blaming the fever on your baby's teething.

The first teeth to erupt are the lower (mandibular) incisors, followed by the upper (maxillary) incisors, then lateral incisors, canine, first molars, and second molars. Female babies usually have an earlier eruption than male babies, and Black babies tend to have teeth sooner than White babies. In rare cases, your baby can be born with a tooth, have teeth erupted before 6 months of age, or experience delayed or asymmetric teeth eruption. If the delay surpasses 18–20 months of age, the child should be evaluated by a pediatric dentist. In cases of complete lack of tooth eruption, your pediatrician will consider genetic or systemic diseases and will make the appropriate referrals.

44.   How do I prevent cavities? When do I start brushing my child's teeth? What toothpaste should I use for my child?

This is a common question with a simple answer. The first appointment with the pediatric dentist should be made at 12 months of age. This is also the time when you start using toothpaste (the size of a pea) spread over a soft toothbrush, twice daily for 2 minutes. Parents must assist with teeth brushing until the child is able to tie their shoelaces (a milestone requiring certain dexterity) or 5 years of age.

Tooth brushing is a milestone that requires fine motor skill needed to properly brush one's teeth. Dental caries, also known as cavities, develop when the microbiome in the mouth reacts with carbohydrates (sugars) and initiates digestion. This lowers the acidity and creates a great environment for cavity formation.

Offering milk bottles at bedtime and allowing your child to drink juice from sippy cups (use open cups instead) creates an environment that promotes cavities. The AAP does not recommend juices for the first 12 months of age, and not to exceed 4 ounces between 12–36 months. It is rare to have a hereditary predisposition for cavities. For the most part, the causes are behavioral.

45. **Why is my 1-year-old not making eye contact? Why is my toddler obsessed with lining up their toys, cars, shoes? Why is my toddler covering their ears when we are in noisy spaces like a circus? Could it be autism?**

Autism and its diagnosis have experienced many metamorphoses in the last two decades. It's gone from not being recognized as a diagnosis in many places in the world, to becoming one of the most commonly discussed and researched developmental disorders. Luckily, we live in a century where information is easily accessible.

Parents are aware of the worrisome symptoms of autism. They notice a lack of eye contact, speech delay, lack of crying when vaccines are administered, and awkwardness in social situations. The child may seem to be too quiet or not cuddly or play by themselves, they have disturbed sleep, and they cover their ears when around loud noises. With food, they could be refusing solids and showing preferences for specific food textures. Regarding what they wear, they may seem uncomfortable with certain clothes, refuse socks or gloves, and prefer only one color and style of clothing. They may dislike being touched or hugged, keep toys aligned, and engage in repetitive behaviors like rocking or hand flapping. They may have an unusually strong preoccupation with parts of toys, a strong mechanical interest in things like trains, cars, ceiling fans, and subway lines. These symptoms of autism spectrum disorder (ASD) are the most common red flags and parents' concerns that are brought to my attention.

I use a few diagnostic tools when I confirm the diagnosis of ASD. One of the most common is the CARS-2 (Childhood Autism Rating Scale, second edition) standard version. This diagnostic instrument is suitable for children under the age of 2 years.

The approach for a child with ASD and their parents is delicate and complex. A team of specialists who craft the EIP (early intervention program) often include a geneticist, developmental specialist, neurologist, and psychiatrist. The sooner the diagnosis is made, the better the chances for improvement.

Your pediatrician will be your best advisor on the step-by-step approach, special schools, and therapies for your child. I have been so blessed to watch many of my ASD kids improve, become self-dependent, and graduate from college.

Pediatrics is a positively charged specialty. The children are like flowers, they need to be watered if they are to grow. We water them with care, love, and patience. Children are the best patients one can ever ask for. They keep you laughing, their honesty is overwhelming, and they act like small stand-up comedians. My pediatric office is always full of surprises!

Did you know that the reason that kids on the autism spectrum tend to hold their ears or need noise-canceling headphones is that their brains can interpret noise as pain? This extreme sound sensitivity is called "hyperacusis." And it can be as rough on them when they hear a person chewing food as when they hear a high-pitched noise. It's important to be aware of the intensity of sounds for your child if they are on the spectrum, as is teaching them to advocate for their needs if they are overwhelmed and need a moment apart from the group and the noise.

46. What should I do if my child is banging their head on the wall?

Although head banging can be seen in children with ASD (autism spectrum disorder) and other developmental problems, it is a part of behavior that is considered normal, although unusual. This is more commonly seen in boys than girls, ages 2–5 years. This is a way of taking out frustration or anxiety, part of a tantrum, or a result of inhibited emotions. For the child, self-harming can feel like it provides some comfort or relief from difficult emotions. Parents may be worried and confused as most of the information they find online regarding self-harm in the form of children banging their heads leads to the diagnosis of ASD.

Once I complete my exam and diagnostic questionnaires and confirm the benign nature of the head-banging behavior, the best advice I can give to parents is to protect their child during the episodes. Parents can also distract them by shifting their attention to a desirable and fun activity, like reading a book, playing with toys, watching a cartoon, taking a walk, or playing with the family pet. Children tend to outgrow this behavior around

4–5 years of age, unless there is an underlying developmental issue.

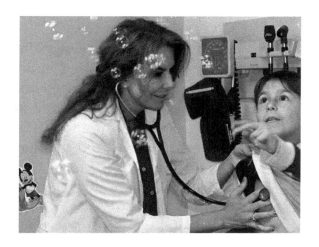

Dr. Daniela Distracting a Child with Bubbles in Her Office

47. Is it normal that my 5-year-old is writing numbers and letters backward?

The parents of my patients love to brag about the reading skills of their children. My patients claim things such as, "They are only 18 months and already recognize some letters." "My girl is 7 and already finished all of the Harry Potter books."

"We started using visual cards to teach my 12-month-old how to read.'" "My 1st grader is reading at the level of a 5th grader." Comments like these melt my heart.

I notice that the children who eventually become avid readers in life were raised in families where parents introduced and encouraged books at an early age, limiting screen time to none for the first 2 years of life. Lack of exposure to books, lack of instruction, neglect, poverty, and low parental education are some of the reasons for children to experience delays with reading.

But what if the child is writing letters and numbers backward or upside-down (mirroring)? Or if they don't recognize simple words or spell them correctly? This is normal until the age of 7–8, but if it persists, it could be a sign of dyslexia. Bring it to your pediatrician's attention, but do not worry, because it is quite common and it rarely persists beyond 8 years of age. It could be due to poor memory or visual processing issues. Letters like b, d, p, and q and numbers like 5 or 3 could be easily confused by young children.

My daughter was mirroring the numbers 5 and 3 until she was 8 years old. My son learned the alphabet at 3, and then he regressed for a short period of time only to quickly pick up his pace again during 1st grade.

Every child is different; every human being has their own learning profile and learning style. Patience and support is the key. My daughter made it to a pre-med college program on a full-ride Division 1 tennis scholarship. My son is thriving in his honor roll high school program and is preparing his applications for pre-med programs at universities. I am sharing this as an example of later success, regardless of the pace of early growth development.

48. Is it normal if my 5-year-old is still wetting the bed?

Approximately 15% of children under the age of 5 wet the bed at night. The medical term doctors use for this condition is "enuresis," which is only diagnosed if bedwetting persists after the age of 5. It is a common, and for the most part, benign condition that children outgrow. By the age of 15 years, only 1–2% will still experience bedwetting. It is frustrating and tiring for parents to deal with night bedwetting.

Bladder dysfunction, neurological diseases, and constipation could be underlying causes and should be considered during diagnosis. Rarely, the condition would be present during the day (diurnal enuresis) versus nocturnal enuresis (nighttime bedwetting). Daytime accidents would need further investigation and referral to an urologist.

Many parents look for answers on how to deal with bedwetting. My best advice to them is to use a mattress protector, distribute the daily fluids intake by offering 40% of the daily requirements in the morning, the other 40% between 12–5 pm, and then leave 20% for the hours before bedtime. Restricting fluids before bedtime could be confusing for some parents, because they could leave the child dehydrated. Make sure that your children are hydrated during the rest of the day!

Using the bathroom before bedtime is important, but waking your child up 2–3 hours after falling asleep has not proved to be beneficial based on the latest AAP recommendations and research. Using a bedwetting alarm, though, is one way of helping your child with nocturnal enuresis. In the case of an accident, the alarm is activated. If the child does not wake up, the parent should wake them up and walk them to the bathroom. By repeating this ritual every night, the child develops a reflex and makes a subconscious connection between the sound of the alarm, waking up, and using the bathroom.

If there are no results in 6 months, the child could be placed on medications. If enuresis is left untreated and neglected, it can lead to psychological disturbances and interfere with their social life, camping, and sleepovers, while causing low self-esteem. Fortunately, most children outgrow bedwetting.

49. When is the right time to start toilet training?

Every pediatrician has encountered multiple questions about potty training. "When is the best time to start teaching my child how to use a toilet? "Doc, can you give me some tips?" "Why is my toddler afraid of the toilet seat and refuses to use it?"

The truth is that toilet training has evolved over the last century. In the early 1900s, the child was treated as a passive participant in the process of toilet training using rigid scheduling, and in 1929, *Parents Magazine* wrote that most healthy babies could be trained by 8 weeks of age ... no, that was not a typo! In the 1940s, Dr. Benjamin Spock began to advocate that parents and caregivers should start potty training only after they observed signs of developmental readiness in their children. He believed that rushed training and rigid scheduling could be harmful and lead to behavioral problems later in life. Spock was influenced by Freud's work about psychological disturbances associated with forceful and rigid toilet training.

Toilet training varies in different cultures. Did you know that the Digo people in East Africa begin toilet training in the first weeks after birth by reading specific cues and behaviors in the baby, and they achieve successful toilet readiness by 4–5 months of age?

Before the invention of the diaper in the 1950s, people used cloth diapers or long ropes and no diapers at all. Babies were swaddled, and the diaper cloth was changed throughout the day.

Today, pediatricians advocate starting the process when the child is psychologically, behaviorally, and developmentally ready. The toilet training process should be fun and less stressful for the child.

Developmentally, the child should be ready at the time of the initiation of the process. The child should be able to walk, be sitting stably, be able to remain dry for a few hours, show an ability to imitate behaviors, demonstrate independence by saying "no," have a desire to please, and show control of functions of elimination.

Daytime bladder control readiness always comes first, and offering the potty after napping and bedtime is the initial step toward toilet training. Nighttime bladder control is achieved the latest, and bowel control comes usually simultaneously with daytime control.

Children also become aware of accidents by 15 months and start pointing and calling for attention to their soiled diapers by 18 to 24 months. By 30–36 months, most children will ask to be taken to the toilet for elimination, and a full pattern of elimination is achieved on average by 48 months.

Potty training has to be delayed if there are major changes in the family dynamics like a caregiver starting a job, moving to a new home, a divorce, or if the mom is expecting a new child.

Toilet training must be approached in a positive way, without punishment and negative reinforcement. Boys should be taught how to urinate first in a sitting position. Training pants are recommended in the transitional stage. Nighttime diapers are advisable until the child fully achieves daytime dryness. The whole process in a cognitively and developmentally ready child takes about 4–6 months.

Dr. Daniela's tips for toilet training:

- Recognize your child's cues and toileting patterns.
- Increase the fluid intake so you can expect more frequent urinary urgency and open opportunities for toilet use.
- Use positive reinforcement.
- Use body language and gestures, sign language, and pictures.
- Schedule bathroom visits based on your child's already built and recognizable patterns.

CHAPTER THREE: BEHAVIORS AND EMOTIONS

Dr. Shellie's Mom Memories of Behaviors and Emotions

As a former assistant principal of a school with over 200 children who had such severe emotional and behavioral needs that they couldn't be in the regular public school, I went into parenthood knowing the extreme sides of behaviors and how to teach coping skills. Even with the less severe versions of what I witnessed with my own children from fears to impulse control issues, it is helpful to know some strategies to cope with emotions and behaviors.

From the age of birth to 5, dealing with the fears of a child is important. For example, as a toddler, Alyssa was terrified of worms. She would explain her nightmares about "wormies" and get very emotional when she saw them on our nature walks or when playing in our backyard. Both Jacob and Alyssa had fears that I wouldn't come back after work, and this is why I wrote my children's book Hopping Off on A Business Trip *which my young daughter illustrated. It tells the story of a mommy kangaroo who hops around the world speaking on stages, and she always comes back home to her joeys! Telling stories to my children has always been a way that I have soothed their minds and explained their world around them in words they could understand.*

Jacob showed very early signs of ADHD, and we needed to redirect him and refocus him on activities often. He was (and still is) fidgety and he can definitely lack impulse control. He struggles with his "executive functioning," which is the ability to display self-control, stay focused despite distractions, plan ahead, meet goals, and follow multiple-step directions even when interrupted.

He's the kind of kid who will simply do whatever his mind says he should do without the little voice in his head telling him to think about it first. We have worked with him on this over the

124

years but as a young child, it meant an adult had to have an eye on him at all times. Incorporating physical activities such as horseback therapy, martial arts, and baseball was important to him when he was young.

Jacob's emotions were difficult to manage when he was little as well. He was quick to anger and often got frustrated. We learned that he needed to have ways of expressing how he was feeling, I had a stop light system for him, and he could tell me when he was feeling green (all good), yellow (he felt like he was getting emotional), and red (he had lost control of the emotion or his impulses got away from him). When Jacob was "on red" he needed to step away from the situation, be redirected, go for a walk, or talk it out with a trusted adult.

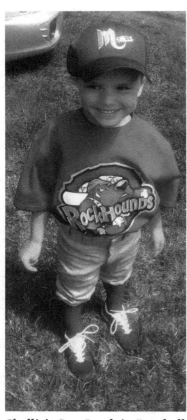

Shellie's Son Jacob in Baseball Uniform

As I'm reflecting on these basic coping strategies, I'm amazed! Jacob is now 14, and he has noticed that I have been working so hard on this book and not getting a lot of sleep. Jacob is actually using those very same "on red" techniques on me as the distracted mom that I taught him at the age of 4. He redirected me by encouraging me to take a nature walk around a local lake with him to step away from the work. Just an hour ago, he told me that I looked too stressed out by my book deadline (yes, I would have been considered "on red" by the old stop light technique). He literally told me to meditate and that he had switched over the laundry from the washer to the dryer for me because he wanted me to step away from it for a moment and "chill out." There is no doubt in my mind that by teaching our kids coping skills at a young age, they will grow into teens and adults who are better equipped for their futures.

If you have any concerns about self-soothing habits such as nail biting or thumb sucking, Dr. Daniela addresses these concerns and more in this important chapter on your child's behaviors and emotions.

Dr. Daniela's Pediatric Prescription for Behavior and Emotions

50. What should I do if my 5-year-old can't sit still in school?

ADHD or attention-deficit/hyperactivity disorder is a troublesome diagnosis for caregivers, teachers, and parents. Signs of hyperactivity are seen as early as preschool age. Being fidgety, impulsive, throwing tantrums for a long period of time, not being able to stay focused for more than a couple of minutes, constantly moving from one activity to another, and being disobedient and aggressive with their play or toward siblings are some of the commonly recognized symptoms of this disorder. Children with ADHD often sleep poorly: their sleep is often interrupted and short. Young children with ADHD can have reckless and impulsive behaviors that could even threaten their lives—for instance, if they run away from the parents on a playground, while crossing the street, or if they escape from the house without the parents knowing.

ADHD could present the symptoms of hyperactivity, attention deficit, or both. Diagnosing the condition early and initiating therapy is key, as it determines how the child under treatment will be able to further adjust to the family and school environment. Behavioral therapy, cognitive therapy, and psychological intervention are the initial steps of approaching ADHD. Medications should be the last resort and are mainly reserved for school-aged children who are falling behind their peers due to distracted behaviors; it's important that they keep their grades at a level of achievement that matches their intelligence. However, like we wouldn't take away a child's glasses in a classroom if they were vision impaired, it is important to provide the tools that our children need to be successful in the classroom, and for some, that may mean they need medication. Remember that all children are individuals and should be treated as such through interventions and accommodations.

ADHD often coexists with other issues such as anxiety, panic disorders, and oppositional defiant disorder. Motor tics are commonly seen in children with ADHD. Other consequences are learning disabilities and comprehension deficits as a result of a lack of focus.

Many parents may wonder why their child has ADHD. Alcohol, smoking, and drug use during pregnancy could be the reason behind an ADHD diagnosis in children. Also, ADHD can be inherited.

A professional team of doctors, including your pediatrician, neurologist, psychiatrist, and developmental specialist works together to make a diagnosis. The teachers work in collaboration with the physicians, because they observe the child's behavior during school hours.

The best tip for my parents whose children have mild cases of ADHD is to find hobbies and sports their children are passionate about and redirect their energy into healthy and enjoyable activities that help them refocus and improve their sleep.

51. Why does my 3-year-old refuse to talk to strangers outside of home? Should I be concerned if my child acts normally at home but appears to be "deaf and mute" in school or with strangers? How can I help support my child?

Is this a case of extreme shyness or selective mutism? Parents are subjective when it comes to their children's personalities. They can say things like their child "is just too shy, like their dad." But the line between being extremely shy and the diagnosis of selective mutism is very fine. Some of the red flags are "My child freezes up around strangers," "My child is not waving or saying hello to other children," "My child is a happy normal, active, and energetic kid at home, fully fluent in their language, but when we leave the house and meet other people (peers or adults) they freeze," or "My child did not say a single word during the whole year of pre-K."

Selective mutism is not an uncommon diagnosis, but we as pediatricians are sometimes guilty of rushing our patients, focusing on growth parameters, blood work, and vaccine administration. Plus, the "Covid Generation" of infants and toddlers had no opportunity to develop their social skills. They may have been raised in a "bubble," which could have caused delays in speech and motor development, as well as social interactions.

Asking the parents how their child(ren) behave in the house and when out, in school, visiting friends and family, or attending after school activities is an important part of the physical exam initial history evaluation.

My son Daniel was 3 years old when I noticed that he would start blinking when we were out dining or when he went to his music and tennis lessons. He was anxious and developed motor tics as a result of it, but the worst was his fear of speaking in public. He would freeze and refuse to communicate even with gestures or using body language. He started playing tennis at the age of 4, and his first lesson was at the USTA National Tennis Center in New York. The venue is massive, and at that time, I had no idea he was showing signs of Selective Mutism. He would freeze, and the coaches had to pick him up and run with him for the drills and tennis games. He did not say a word for an entire year in preschool. On the last day of the school year, the teachers hugged him and he whispered "bye"—this was the first word he verbalized in public. His teacher burst into tears of joy. Soon after, I reached out to the Child Mind Institute in Manhattan, where, with the help of a psychologist, Daniel found his voice and broke his fears of speaking in public.

Selective mutism, when diagnosed early, is most often successfully treated. Cognitive behavioral therapy (CBT), play therapy, and exposure to social situations are among some of the most successful methods of therapy. Helping children with selective mutism find their voices is critical for their future development, social interactions, and adaptation to their environment.

If you notice that your child is exceptionally shy, please talk to your pediatrician. Children tend to have no inhibitions. Shyness could be a personality trait, but when it becomes a part of a diagnosis, it needs to be addressed and treated. If therapy is initiated before the age of 7, the results have better outcomes.

52. Why isn't my child showing emotion? Why don't they like to be hugged? Why don't they smile?

When you have a crying and fussy baby at home it can be overwhelming and frustrating. The sleep deprivation, the worries of why your baby is in discomfort and crying, doubting yourself, and wondering why you can't calm your baby leads to questions with no answers, frustration, and desperation. Most babies are fussy for various reasons (e.g., they are colicky, have a rash, or they are hungry), but if your baby is too quiet, not smiling, not responding to noises, refusing to cuddle and be touched, and not crying during vaccine administrations and blood draws, these are all red flags. They could be the first signs of hearing loss (isolated or as part of genetic disease) or even autism.

It is natural for humans to seek love, care, and cuddles. Address your concerns, and share them with your pediatrician. Your baby will require a full developmental screening and perhaps genetic and metabolic testing.

Even though hearing tests are done upon discharge from the hospital nursery, hearing deficits could be missed. Delivering your baby at home is becoming more common, so not all newborns are tested in the first 24–48 hours of life.

Babies are born with personalities, and just because they are small and fully dependent on their parents does not mean that they are emotionless. Tune into your child's needs from the beginning.

53. Why is my child biting their nails, pulling their hair, and biting their cuticles?

Nail biting is a self-soothing behavior in moments of stress and anxiety that leads to a bad habit. Finger and toenail or cuticle biting, and

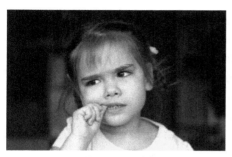

Nail Biting Habit

pulling and eating hair, are some of the most commonly seen "bad habits" in my little and my not-so-little patients. Bad habits can be triggered by insecurities, fears, and anxieties or part of obsessive-compulsive disorders (OCD). Children find ways to soothe themselves, from the teething baby biting on their fist to the preschooler who fights separation anxiety, there are many reasons your baby or child can experience feeling insecure and anxious.

The bad news is that this self-soothing activity can quickly become a bad habit. It takes self-control and mindfulness to combat this which can be foreign to most young children. Nail and cuticle biting is seen in 30% of children older than 7 years and 45% of teens. The anxiety can become so severe that some kids under stress curl up and bite their toenails. The constant self-inflicted damage to the nails leads to the destruction and shortening of the nail matrix. I have heard of some cases where a baby is born with nail plate structure malformation due to thumb sucking in the womb.

Hair pulling is also known as trichotillomania (TTM), and it is a disorder characterized by an uncontrollable urge to pull out one's own hair during mounting tension. The hair pulling tends to be followed by a sense of relief. Bald spots on the scalp area could lead to the diagnosis.

If this is in combination with pica—a condition in which the child is eating things such as hair that are not supposed to be digested— it can lead to bezoar formations, which are clumps of the non-

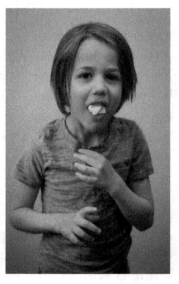

Child with Pica Eating Paper

digestible materials in the stomach that can cause severe intestinal obstruction.

Skin picking is another behavior that may cause skin infections. Cognitive behavioral therapies combined with family and child psychotherapy must be considered with such behaviors.

54. What should I do if my young child is masturbating?

Masturbation is a commonly observed behavior after the age of 2, when children start exploring their bodies, and they discover that touching or rubbing their private parts is associated with pleasure and self-comfort. They use their fingers or hands or rub their genitals against furniture or other objects. Masturbation rarely requires further evaluation or follow-up unless it becomes an obsession where the repetitiveness of the behavior can cause infections and self-inflicted trauma or if the child is masturbating in public. Once the behavior has been noticed by parents, they usually bring it to the attention of their pediatrician.

A child may masturbate as often as several times a day or just once a week. Masturbation occurs when a child is bored, sleepy, watching TV, or under stress. There is no medical cause for this behavior. Negative reinforcement and time out can only make it seem dirty or wicked and cause emotional harm or feelings of shame, guilt, and sexual hang-ups. Teaching your child about their bodies by using appropriate books, videos, and other educational materials can help them understand their bodies better. Once your child discovers masturbation, they seldom stop doing it completely, but around the age of 5–6, they become more sensitive and learn to do it discreetly and privately.

This is a common question that I get from my parents. Many parents want to know how to be the perfect caretaker for their child and what is considered "normal." They want to know how they should approach this "perverse behavior" or "bad habit" and if there is a need for the support of a psychologist.

The way to handle masturbation is to first understand that it is impossible to eliminate it. The

140

only thing parents can control is where the children do it. A reasonable goal is to permit it in the home bathroom and in the bedroom. Distract and discipline your child if masturbation occurs in other places by explaining to them, "I understand that this makes you feel good and it's ok to do it in your bedroom or in the bathroom, but not in front of other people or other places." Talk to your child's teachers and inform them about the concerns and limitations you have discussed with your child. Never label masturbation as evil, sinful, or dirty. Do not restrain their hands because this could lead to resistance, and sexual inhibitions later in life.

Professional help is needed if your child continues to do it in front of other people or tries to touch others inappropriately or if you suspect they were taught to do it by someone else or you feel your child is deeply unhappy or under stress.

55. Why won't my child stop sucking on their thumb?

Thumb sucking is a self-soothing behavior that occurs as a primitive reflex, is observed in early childhood, and for the most part is outgrown after 6 years of age. There are no apparent causative factors, but thumb sucking becomes a habit that is difficult to break if it persists after 5–6 years of age.

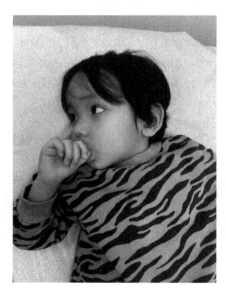

Child Sucking Thumb

Thumb guards and positive reinforcement are the most appropriate approaches to deal with the habit. This behavior is self-limited and unless it becomes chronic has no associated side effects. The persistence of thumb sucking, however, could cause paronychia or infection of the thumbnail bed requiring antibiotics, misalignment of the teeth, and deformities of the mouth. The prolonged presence of the thumb in the mouth creates pressure against the developing jaw and teeth. The complications seen with persistent thumb sucking are delayed or abrupt eruption of the teeth and malformations like anterior open bite, high and narrow arch palate, posterior crossbite, or a temporomandibular joint (where your jaw attaches to the skull) disorder. With the help of a pediatric dentist and your pediatrician, the thumb-sucking habit can be controlled.

56. Why did my child start wetting the bed and asking for a baby bottle after we brought home a new baby?

Regression of an older sibling after the family welcomes a newborn is indeed very common. The sibling or siblings who had all the attention from their parents suddenly have to share it with a new family member. The newborn requires 24/7 supervision and care and the older siblings suddenly have to adapt to the new dynamics and the changed environment. If there is more than one sibling, regression is less often observed. Noticing your older one bedwetting after being toilet trained, asking for a baby bottle, or intending to breastfeed are among the most observed behaviors. Sometimes older children experience difficulties falling asleep and ask to be cuddled like babies.

Allowing mom to rest for the newborn and spending time with the other children should be reinforced. A healthy parental relationship is indeed critical to help your children deal with the new situation. It can be helpful to have a hands-on partner or helper to take the children out for a walk, share activities with them, and find ways to keep them busy and entertained.

57.Why does my child grind their teeth at night?

Grinding the teeth at night is known to be associated with parasite infestation in many developing countries. In fact, this is a myth. Children are unaware of the grinding, also known as bruxism. Bruxism involves activation of the masticatory (chewing) muscles and results in grinding during sleep and teeth clenching. The grinding of the teeth tends to peak around the ages of 3 to 6 years; however, grinding can happen throughout a person's life due to stress. Some associations with teeth grinding, OSA (obstructive sleep apnea), snoring, and nasal congestion have been made. Children with ADHD, anxiety, and sleep disorders, like sleepwalking, enuresis, and nightmares have been shown to experience teeth grinding more often. No mouth guards are recommended or used in children. Tooth enamel damage or wear has rarely been reported. Morning tenderness of the jaw muscles or headaches could be present. If persistent and troublesome, then bruxism may need an intervention. Talk to your dentist or pediatrician.

58. How do I handle my child's fears?

Fears are unpleasant emotions in response to real or imaginary danger. The brain circuits in the amygdala (the part of the brain involved with the experiences of emotions) get stimulated and send signals to the body and mind in preparation for danger. This will trigger the "flight, fight, freeze, and fawn" responses as your child reacts to the danger; they will run away, cry, close their eyes, look for support from the parents, and/or hide.

The fear response is an important brain function that helps humans survive, but if it is dysfunctional, overly stimulated, or irrational, it can become a pathology that needs to be addressed and treated—this is when a FEAR becomes a PHOBIA. Phobias are irrational fears that do not respond to reassurance. Some of the underlying causes leading to phobias include: children with generalized anxieties; those who are living in dysfunctional and/or abusive families, poverty, or neglect.

Fears in early childhood tend to be more of a result of neuronal mirroring or mimicking and adapting the fears of the parents. Fears of falling, fears of darkness, and loud noises are primitive instincts and normal reactions of children between 0–2 years of age. The brain develops from the bottom to the top: think of a tree or a plant that develops from a seed, grows roots, and then follows with the trunk and branches. If we simplify the brain's development, it starts with the brainstem (responsible for breathing, detecting hunger, consciousness, blood pressure, and heart rate), followed by the limbic system (responsible for emotions like anger, laughter, crying, and behaviors needed for survival, like the fight and flight responses), and then the prefrontal cortex, which plays a role in decisions making, impulse inhibition, attention, memory, and control. The brain actually isn't fully developed until around 25 years of age.

Do not blame your toddler for not listening to you when they run out in the street chasing their ball. Their prefrontal cortex is way too immature to provide self-protection and self-defense mechanisms. Of course, we still need to correct and redirect the child in dangerous situations. Attempt to help your child confront their fears when appropriate and seek therapeutic support if the fears are turning into irrational phobias.

CHAPTER FOUR: INJURIES

Dr. Shellie's Mom Memories of Injuries

My children are teens now, but I have definitely had my fair share of emergency room visits and needing to call their Uncle John, who runs Grand Avenue Urgent Care in Wyoming for what to do when they are injured! So if you don't have a great nurse on speed dial like I do, you will want to have this chapter of The Prescription for a Happy and Healthy Child *handy for those inevitable injuries occur. From my daughter as a toddler accidentally breaking her leg falling off of a bouncy slide, to my son severing his pinky finger's tendon, I have had my fair share of scary moments and the "mom guilt" that tends to follow when kids get hurt!*

One summer as a teen, I was a counselor at a burn unit camp, so the question in this chapter that deals with burns and how to react is so important to me! If some of the parents of the campers had known more about burn prevention or if they had a fire extinguisher in the home, some of those kids would have a different story of scarring and healing.

Whether your child steps on a rusty nail accidentally or if you see that they accidentally ate something that is inedible, you need to know what to do, and reaction time is important. Know that injuries will happen in your child's lifetime, but prepare yourself with what you should do when they occur.

Dr. Daniela's Pediatric Prescription for Injuries

59. What should I do if I cut my baby's or child's nails and they start bleeding?

My patients' parents will always hear me emphasizing the importance of filing or gently cutting the fingernails of their newborns. There is no need to use baby mittens, as they can create a humid environment which benefits the growth of fungus and causes skin infections and atopic dermatitis or eczema. If the mittens are too loose, they may become a choking hazard for your baby. Keep the hands open and free, and file the nails or cut them. Your newborn will be exploring different parts of their bodies, and if left with long nails, they may scratch their face and (rarely) their eyes.

I will never forget the frustration of the mother of a patient of mine whose newborn was inconsolable crying for hours, and after several visits to ER and ruling out organic causes for the crying, I decided to perform a fluorescein test of the scleras of the eyes, only to diagnose a superficial corneal abrasion that was causing irritation and eye pain. It was self-inflicted by the baby, who scratched the cornea of their eye with their fingernails.

How do you trim the baby's nails? Use daylight, ask for someone else to help, and hold the baby. Separate the finger pad from the nail to avoid cutting the skin. Cut the nails on the fingers and toes straight across to avoid ingrown nails. If you accidentally cut the skin, apply immediate pressure to stop the bleeding. Clean the area with water and soap, and use an alcohol pad to sanitize the area. The most important preventive measure when taking care of the baby's nails is to use a clean and sterile nail clipper and/or filer. Your baby is not fully-immunized, so to avoid infection, you have to use a new and sterile clipper.

60. What should I do if my older child pokes my toddler in the eye, hand, or leg?

Intentional or unintentional eye poking by pen or pencil is not uncommon, but it is always an emergency when it leads to an eye injury. Your child needs to be seen by an ophthalmologist, and the best advice would be to call the emergency number in your town or drive your injured child to the nearest ER.

Poking the skin with a pencil depending on the depth of the wound may also need to be evaluated by a doctor. The tip of the pencil is made out of clay and graphite (not lead). Although it's a common concern of parents, you can't get lead poisoning from being poked by one because pencils do not contain lead. Lead styles of pens and pencils were used by the Ancient Romans centuries ago, but in the 1500s a large deposit of graphite was discovered in England and was used for pencils. After that, people confused graphite with lead.

61. How do I stop a nosebleed?

Young children tend to pick at their noses, and as a result of this constant irritation and trauma to the area, the nose can bleed. Parents must be encouraged to cut the nails of their children on a regular basis, especially if they have the habit of picking at their noses.

The inner parts of the nostrils have a vascular network of 5 arteries that can easily bleed under trauma. The trauma could be self-inflicted, by picking with fingernails, or as a result of trauma during sports or car accidents. Common colds and constant nasal congestion are other reasons blood vessel walls may become thin and start bleeding.

To stop a nosebleed, parents and older children should gently press just above the soft part of the nostrils in the middle of the nasal bridge for approximately 3–5 minutes. Parents can even teach their children how to properly apply pressure over the nasal bridge. It should not take more than 5 minutes to control the bleeding. There is no need to ask your child to lie down or keep their head and chin up and bend the head backward. If your child is old enough to blow their nose on their own, ask them to blow their nose gently, but only after the acute bleeding has been controlled. If there are blood clots left, they will cause continuous bleeding. If the bleeding doesn't stop within 5 minutes, call your pediatrician as there could be an underlying bleeding disorder that needs to be further investigated. Ice packs over the nasal

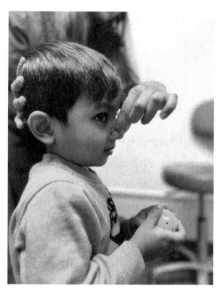
Apply Pressure for a Nosebleed

bridge may help the blood vessels constrict and slow the bleeding. Vasoconstrictive topical medications could be used by your pediatrician to control the bleeding. If there is severe nasal trauma with nasal septum deviation (if the nose looks crooked), you need to see a maxillofacial surgeon immediately.

62. What do I do if my baby falls off the bed?

First, never leave your infant or toddler unattended. But if they do get hurt, every fall requires immediate attention. The most common falls are from the bed, crib, chairs, and of course monkey bars. Every doctor will ask if the child cried immediately after, if they lost consciousness, and if they have vomited since the fall. Other questions they will ask include:

- Were they confused or convulsing after the fall?
- What was the height the child fell from?
- What was the surface the child landed on after the fall?
- Are there obvious skull, face, or other bone deformities?

If there was loss of consciousness you MUST call 911 or emergency services in your area ASAP. A parent is never supposed to watch the child after a fall without having professional advice and medical evaluation. Falls could lead to serious brain injuries and can be lethal. Head injuries could cause skull fractures and/or brain hemorrhaging which could lead to life-threatening blood loss. Falls from monkey bars and playgrounds are the most common reasons for ER visits.

Do not underestimate the extent of the injury, even without any loss of consciousness and obvious deformities or symptoms. Call your pediatrician or visit the nearest ER.

63. How should I handle an injury from a rusty nail?

Plantar puncture wounds (on the feet), especially caused by a rusty nail need to be evaluated and treated immediately. In the United States, most children are fully immunized, and because of this, they have passive immunity against tetanus, which could be contracted from a wound from rusted metal. Sadly, 1 in 5 children internationally do not have access to essential immunizations including tetanus.

In the case of rusty nails, the most common bacterial infection is caused by *Pseudomonas aeruginosa*. It is treatable if the appropriate antibiotics are prescribed. Cleaning the wound with iodine solution or any other antiseptic solution is the first step to treat such wounds. X-rays and other imaging studies should also be considered for examining the wound for small parts of the foreign body that may have broken off inside the wound. Based on the immunization status of the child or the wound type (clean versus dirty) the ER physician will determine if a tetanus vaccination or tetanus immunoglobulins will be administered.

Tennis shoe puncture wounds, where a nail goes through the shoe and into the foot, are associated with infections from *Pseudomonas aeruginosa*. *Staphylococcus aureus* and beta-hemolytic streptococcus. If left unattended the puncture wounds can lead to serious complications like soft tissue necrosis (death of the tissue), skin infection or cellulitis, skin abscess, and osteomyelitis (an infection of the bone).

In warm countries where children run barefoot, puncture wounds are commonly seen throughout the year. The proper steps to approach a puncture wound are:

- Seek help immediately.
- Clean properly.

- Remove any remaining foreign bodies.
- Treat the wound.

64. How should I handle accidental burns? What about superglue incidents?

Burns are painful injuries, and for the most part, they are unintentional and accidental in origin. Parents are overwhelmed with multitasking. So many times, I have heard stories like, "My child was running around, and they accidentally dumped a hot cup of coffee or boiled water over their face and body." Accidental burns can occur after spilling hot liquids over the child's skin, by children using lighters, or by the child getting too close to an unattended stove. Less common causes of burns include not checking the water temperature in the bathtub before bathing your baby or failing to install a faucet spout cover to prevent your child from reaching the hot water tap. These are easily preventable with the proper childproofing products.

Childproof against water burns by using anti-scalding devices for faucets and shower heads and setting your hot water temperature to 120°F or 48.8°C on your water heater. Old radiators in a home can be child proofed by using a guard or isolating them with a safety gate.

Wax burns are devastating and difficult to treat; they can leave severe scarring and deformities. Burns are thermal injuries that cause irreversible skin tissue destruction. The burn triggers a cascade of reactions on a cellular level, involving the release of vasoactive mediators like oxygen radicals, prostaglandins, and cytokines. In children, burns affecting more than 15% of the total body surface area (TBSA) can result in systemic reactions requiring hospitalization for IV hydration and pain management.

One of the most devastating wax burns I have ever seen was caused by wax spilled over the face which left the child blind. All parents, but especially first-time parents need to be educated on child safety and counseled on injury prevention.

The initial treatment of isolated, minor thermal injuries consists mainly of removing clothing and debris, cooling, and simple cleansing with water and soap. The injury should be wrapped with appropriate skin dressing, and after being examined and assessed by the pediatrician, pain management and preventative tetanus shots will be considered.

First-degree burns leave only mild redness. If offset with a cold water rinse right after the accident, a first-degree burn should heal fully.

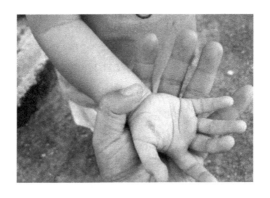

First-Degree Burn

Second-degree burns form blisters. Popping or manipulating the bleb (blister) can cause infection, so it's best to leave them as is.

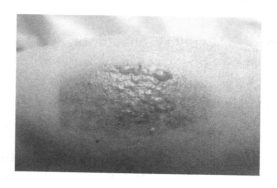

Second-Degree Burn

Third-degree burns are deep and cause permanent damage to the skin with not only keloid scarring, but loss of innervation and sensitivity of the area.

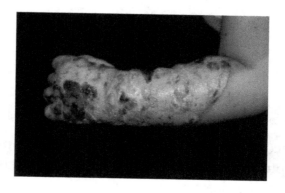

Third-Degree Burn

Regardless of the burn location, a detailed history should be taken by the pediatrician to rule out possible child abuse. If you are sharing custody with your partner and notice a burn on their body, call your pediatrician to discuss it. Scalding burns that have a sharply demarcated edge, burns in the distinct shape of an object, small circular burns matching a cigarette or cigar tip, burns on the perineal area (the area of skin between genitals such as the vaginal opening or scrotum and anus) matching a "dip-in" pattern (e.g., child dipped into scalding water) all raise suspicions about physical abuse.

Regardless of the burns and their cause, place your child in a safe area and rinse the burned area with cold, (but not freezing cold water) for about 10 minutes. For the face, you can use a wet towel, and if the inside of the mouth is injured you can let your child chew on a piece of ice cube. Remove all tight clothing, jewelry, and belts, especially if they are covering the burned area. Apply petroleum jelly over the affected areas if it is handy. Call your pediatrician, and if the face is involved, proceed to the nearest ER and seek help immediately.

Another thermal injury, frostbite, can be quite damaging when neglected and if the parents are unaware of the danger. Spending only 15 minutes in a temperature colder than negative 15°F or negative 26°C can cause severe frostbite. Winter sports are lots of fun and wonderful outdoor activities, but parents should be cautious.

How to be Cautious with Outdoor Winter Sports

- Check the forecast.
- Wear warm clothes.
- Cover the face, nose, ears, hands, fingers, feet, and toes.
- Use warmers.
- If possible, take time out to warm the children in enclosed areas with a warm cup of hot chocolate and or water.

If you notice the skin turning white, this is the first sign that warming is needed. Bring the child to a temperature-regulated environment ASAP. Remove any wet clothing, and make sure they avoid walking on frostbitten feet (because it increases tissue damage). Do not rewarm frostbitten skin if there is a possibility of refreezing before reaching definitive care in case of severe injury.

If prehospital warming is needed for potential frostbite, the options include placing the affected area in warm (not hot—ideally 98.6°F or 37°C) water or warming it using body heat, or by placing frostbitten fingers in the armpits.

Do not rub frostbitten skin areas in an attempt to rewarm them. This can cause further damage. Avoid the use of stoves or fires to

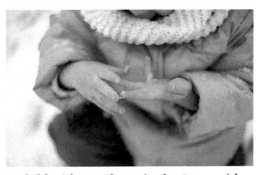

Child without Gloves in the Snow with Frostbite

rewarm frostbitten tissue. Such tissue may be lacking physical sensation, and burns can result.

Winter and snow can bring so much joy to children. Bundle up and let your kids play during the winter season. This will strengthen their immune system and keep them happy and healthy.

Crazy glue accidents also can cause mild burns, but soaking the fingers in warm water immediately after the accident can help with dissolving the glue and removing it from the skin without leaving permanent skin damage. Do not use paper towels or tissues.

65. What should I do if my child steps on broken glass?

It is an all too common scenario of the mom cleaning the kitchen or setting the dinner table and knocking off a glass or plate, which bursts into millions of small pieces. By the time she starts cleaning the floor, their toddler is screaming and pointing to their feet.

I am sure that most people have had a mild or severe injury caused by a broken glass cutting the skin. Most commonly, these injuries are on the soles of the feet or the palms of the hands.

After noticing the injury, remove the visible pieces of glass from the skin. I suggest visiting the ER and receiving an X-ray to make sure there are no foreign bodies left in the skin. After the skin laceration is cleaned and closed, it should be treated with antibiotics as needed, based on the depth and cleanliness of the injury.

66. What do I do if my child swallows a penny, batteries, or a magnet?

As soon as your child starts crawling and walking, safety becomes a priority. Childproof the house, and never leave your baby unattended unless the environment is safe and secure. Sadly, accidents happen quickly and even when all precautions have been taken to provide the safest possible environment because mobile infants and toddlers put everything in their mouths by instinct and out of curiosity.

The most commonly ingested foreign bodies are coins and button batteries from hearing aids, remote controls, game toys, and calculators. Foreign bodies larger than 12 mm in diameter usually get lodged in the esophagus. If they remain there long enough, usually more than 8–12 hours, they can cause ulceration and even perforation of the esophagus, a true and critical emergency. The severity of the damage of the mucous lining of the gastrointestinal (GI) tract depends on the charge load of the battery. Coins can pass through the trachea, but they can also get lodged in there and cause respiratory symptoms, like cough, choking, and drooling. Though it is rare, if a battery is swallowed at the same time as a magnet, they can become trapped in the intestine, causing gut necrosis (death to the tissue) and/or obstruction which becomes an immediate need for surgery.

Be aware of easy access to candies on holidays and especially Halloween. My daughter was 13 months old when she choked on the wrapper of a candy she took from the basket with Halloween treats. I acted quickly and luckily was able to see it and sweep it out of her mouth. This became a terrifying moment even for a pediatrician mom.

If the ingestion of the foreign body is witnessed and results in choking and/or loss of consciousness, the child will require CPR intervention and a 911 call. If the child swallows the foreign body without experiencing any symptoms, an ER visit and urgent examination is still warranted. Imaging studies like X-rays are usually the first step towards properly diagnosing the case and deciding on the intervention and treatment plan. Even if the foreign body has passed the esophagus and is in the stomach or the intestines, the child is asymptomatic, and the physical exam is normal, careful observation would be warranted.

CHAPTER FIVE: COMMON ILLNESSES

Dr. Shellie's Mom Memories of Common Illnesses

Every day, I would walk up to the red door at the daycare that was in a sweet little house near the university where I was a professor. On all my breaks when I didn't have office hours, I would go to the daycare to breastfeed and snuggle my baby. I recall how difficult it was for me to walk away to go back to teaching classes in person but it was a necessity during that time before I became the CEO for Inspiring Lives International and I established my own hours around my children's needs. I say all this because once my children were around other people in daycare and then schools, they were exposed to the germs that caused multiple common illnesses.

From strep throats to ear infections and stomach issues to the common cold ... you name it, we experienced it in my home! Plus, we lived through the pandemic of Covid-19, so I have experienced multiple illnesses with my children. This chapter will help you to comfort your child as they heal up and get well.

Dr. Daniela's Pediatric Prescription for Common Illnesses

67. If my child has a common cold, do they need antibiotics? Why are they getting sick every month?

Common colds are accountable for the majority of sick visits in pediatrics, in the first 5 years of life. Every pediatrician is asked multiple times questions like: "Why is my child sick?" "How did they get sick?" "My child has been coughing for 3 days. Can you prescribe antibiotics, please?" "What medications does my child need?" "Why not antibiotics?"

Being a pediatrician requires lots of patience and incredible listening skills because the vast majority of our specialty is about educating and preventing disease. After all, it is our responsibility to teach the parents what is best for their kids so they can build strong immunity through making healthy choices at a young age. I was lucky enough to grow up on a farm in Bulgaria, where my breakfast was fresh goat or cow milk and boiled eggs from the chickens my grandparents were raising. For snacks, I would pull carrots from the ground or climb on the cherry trees and enjoy the juicy fruits. My patients in New York City are not as lucky as I was as a child to have access to natural and organically fresh foods.

Innate immunity plays an important role in how our bodies handle common colds. Building the microbiome starts at the moment we take our first breath and are welcomed to planet earth. Studies have shown that newborns delivered by C-section lack or have low counts of strains found in the healthy gut, called Bacteroides, which vaginally delivered babies usually have. Research supports the fact that Bacteroides microbes influence the immune system of their hosts and help to fight inflammation.

My goal as a pediatrician is to educate my parents from the moment I meet them during their first consultation visit before delivering the baby. It is important for parents to understand that we as human species have to live with numerous invisible microorganisms, and to build an agreeable co-existence, we have to get to know each other, metaphorically and literally. The reason why we recommend avoidance of crowds in the first 40–60 days of the newborn's life is not because they are unimmunized, but rather we want to minimize exposure to common colds and unnecessary hospital visits and admissions that will require invasive procedures like blood draws, urinary-tract catheterization, and in some cases even lumbar puncture. The immune system of your newborn is still immature and it takes time for it to develop and become able to fight common colds in a predictable manner.

Common colds are caused by viruses like respiratory syncytial virus (RSV), influenza, parainfluenza, adenovirus, coronavirus, SARS-CoV-2, human bocavirus, metapneumovirus, coxsackievirus, enterovirus, and many more. Rhinovirus has at least 100 different strains and is the most commonly seen and diagnosed virus in the months of September to April. The rest of the viruses have more or less stable presentations throughout the fall and winter months.

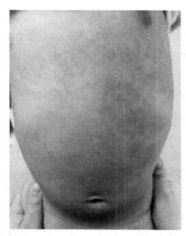

Roseola ("sixth disease" or "three-day fever") is another frequently seen viral illness caused by the B variant of human herpesvirus type 6. It is more prevalent during the spring and fall months and affects children in the age group of 7–24 months presenting with fever for 1–3 days followed by the development of rash right after the fever breaks. Parents seek medical attention twice: first because of the fever and initial cold-like symptoms, and second right after the skin rash erupts.

Roseola Rash on a Child

Common cold viruses produce lasting immunity, but do little to protect or prevent subsequent colds, because there are so many subtypes and they constantly undergo mutation.

Viruses that can cause common colds are spread by three mechanisms. Hand contact (e.g., the infected individual was touching their mouth or nose and they made contact shaking hands) and self-inoculating of one's own conjunctivae (which is the mucous membrane that covers the front of the eye and inside the eyelids) or

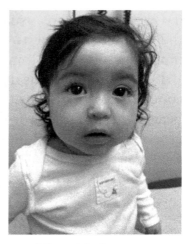

Toddler with the Common Cold Dr. Daniela's Office

nasal mucosa (e.g., touching your nose or eyes and then your mouth and vice versa). Inhalation of small particle droplets that become airborne from coughing and sneezing is another way of transmission. The third mechanism is via deposition of large droplets expelled during coughing or sneezing when they land on the nasal or conjunctival mucosa (this requires close contact with an infected person).

The average incubation period for a cold is 1–2 days; the symptoms usually present on day 3 after the contact and last 10–14 days on average. The most common symptoms of colds are fever above 101°F or 38.5°C, nasal congestion, runny nose, cough, sneezing, chest tightness, muscle aches, headaches, vomiting, or diarrhea. If the symptoms are mainly affecting the upper airways, we will diagnose your child with an upper respiratory infection (URI) from a common cold virus.

On the other hand, if the symptoms are mainly affecting the gastrointestinal tract and present with vomiting, abdominal pain, and/or diarrhea, we call it acute gastroenteritis (AGE) caused by a common cold virus. If we have both URI and AGE, it falls under the diagnosis of a viral syndrome.

The treatment is supportive. Antibiotics do not treat viral infections and antiviral medications are available only against Influenza and SARS-Cov-2 or Covid-19. Antiviral medications are not routinely prescribed to children and not recommended unless the child is immunocompromised or suffers from severe underlying respiratory disease (e.g., asthma or cystic fibrosis).

Controlling the fever and providing the child with comfort is our primary task as pediatricians and caretakers. Hydrating the child with warm drinks and irrigating the sinuses with nasal saline solution to soften the nasal secretions and help with expectoration is the main goal. Using a cool mist humidifier (not warm) can provide some relief as well. Your pediatrician will help you differentiate common colds from seasonal allergies, which present similarly, but the children are typically active and don't have a fever with seasonal allergies.

Over-the-counter medications are not recommended to control the cough for children under the age of 4 years old. If your child requires additional treatment, it will be upon the physical examination and the decision of your pediatrician.

68.   What do I do if my child is exposed to hand, foot, and mouth disease?

Hand, foot, and mouth disease (HFMD) is a clinical syndrome presenting with oral vesicular lesions and maculopapular (red elevated skin lesions) particularly over the hands (palms) and feet (soles). The rest of the body could be affected as well. The syndrome is benign and resolves spontaneously in about 5–7 days. More than 22 types of enteroviruses are involved, with the most common one being coxsackievirus A.

High fever and decreased appetite are the most commonly seen symptoms. The lesions are painful and cause dysphagia (pain on swallowing) which can lead to dehydration. Depending on the viral type, gastrointestinal symptoms could be part of the syndrome. The prevalence of this viral illness is during summer and early autumn months, and it typically affects children 1–5 years of age.

Isolate the infected child from other children while providing comfort by controlling the fever. Offer cool drinks to the child. When I mention the frozen treats like "popsicles" and "ice cream," it's

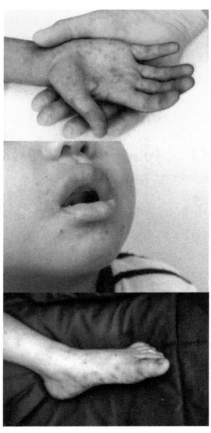

Children with Hand, Foot, and Mouth Disease

like I said magical words, and I get a big smile from the child patient and the parent is surprised by this recommendation. Avoiding acidic and spicy foods is also recommended.

Outbreaks of HFMD occur worldwide involving daycares, summer camps, communities, schools, and hospital wards.

The viruses are transmitted by contact with oral or respiratory secretions, or from person-to-person by the fecal-oral route. The child won't build lifelong immunity against coxsackievirus (which is the leading cause of HFMD) and may have repeated infections throughout the years.

69. What should I do if my child is snoring every night, sleeps with their mouth open and has yellow snot for two weeks and a persistent cough?

Before I get to the pathophysiology of sinus infections, I will give you a short introduction to the face anatomy of the child. Sinuses are 4 pairs of hollow cavities in the face. Maxillary and ethmoid sinuses are present at birth. Maxillary sinuses are next to the nasal cavities and under the cheeks. Ethmoid sinuses are on each side of the nostrils and they communicate with the brain. Sphenoid sinuses are on each side of the temple bones and they form at age 1–2 years. The last ones to form are the frontal sinuses, located behind your forehead and they form around 5–6 years of age and reach adult size around 12 years of age.

All sinuses have small holes that communicate with the nasal airways. They are all covered by a lining called "mucosa," and the top layer of the lining is covered with tiny hairs called "cilia." The cilia trap all foreign bodies, either viruses, microorganisms, dust mites, or gaseous chemicals. Imagine a grass lawn on a windy day. These are the motions of the cilia, and they move the inhaled foreign particles out of the nostrils and the fresh inhaled air that we breathe in (21% oxygen and 79% nitrogen). The mucosal lining heats and humidifies the air that reaches our lungs.

Sinus infections are caused by viruses, and once they start replicating in our nostrils and sinuses, the mucus builds up, and the tissue lining the sinuses swells, preventing adequate air ventilation. The viruses, bacteria, and fungus trapped inside are growing their families by replicating. In acute sinus infection, which is the most commonly seen in children and caused by viral common colds, the symptoms last around 7–14 days. A runny nose with thick yellow or green secretions, fever and headaches, and tenderness over the middle part of the face are the symptoms of acute sinus infection.

Controlling the fever and irrigating the nasal and paranasal cavities (sinuses) is the treatment of choice. By spraying nasal decongestants, like normal saline solution of 0.65%, we "shower" the sinuses and cause constriction of the vessels, which helps the sinuses shrink and open up so the mucus is drained out of them.

Subacute sinus infection lasts 14–30 days, and in chronic sinusitis, the symptoms may persist for up to 90 days. In cases of bacterial overgrowth where the symptoms are not improving and the child has persistent fever and trouble breathing, oral antibiotics will be considered.

70. What should I do if my child has a sore throat?

If I have to talk statistics, in my daily practice more than half of the sick walk-in patients complain of sore throat. When infants and toddlers get feverish and congested, parents would be sharing concerns like, "My baby can't swallow, maybe their throat hurts." A sore throat is a painful sensation in the back of the pharynx (upper throat), accompanied with painful swallowing and discomfort when coughing or drinking liquids and eating solids. A sore throat could be a symptom of a common cold, but in the absence of nasal congestion and runny nose, it could be strep throat or streptococcal pharyngitis.

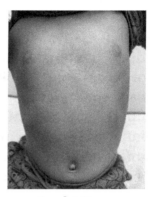

Scarlet Fever Sandpaper Rash over the Trunk

What is strep throat, and why must we diagnose it on time and treat it as soon as

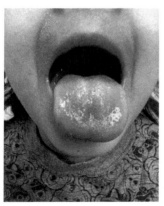

Strawberry Tongue is One of the Classic Signs of Strep Throat Infection

possible? Strep throat is caused by group A streptococcus bacteria (*Streptococcus pyogenes*), and it presents with fever, headaches, abdominal pain, and severe throat pain with or without white exudates (fluid-filled bumps) on the back of the posterior wall. (Note that viral infections and

185

allergies do not present with exudates.) Small red dots or broken vessels on the roof of the mouth are one of the classical symptoms of strep throat. The tip of the tongue has the texture and resemblance of a strawberry, thus called "strawberry tongue." Sandpaper-like papular dots may cover the face, upper arms, and upper trunk as a result of the inflammation and are still part of the streptococcal infection. In this case, your pediatrician will diagnose scarlet fever.

Your pediatrician will prescribe antibiotics that you must comply with and complete as directed. Your child will be able to return to school 24 hours after the initiation of the prescribed antibiotics. Antibiotics seem to eliminate the bacteria from the oral cavity in about 80–90% of cases in the first 24 hours. Treatment will prevent

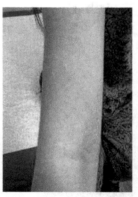

Scarlet Fever Rash as Part of Streptococcal Pharyngitis Infection

complications that can extend beyond the oropharynx (or mouth cavity).

Complicated strep throat can lead to ear infections (otitis media), abscess (pus-like collection) of the tonsils, sinusitis, meningitis (brain infection), and bacteremia (blood infection). Penicillin or Amoxicillin are the antibiotics of choice. There are alternatives if your child is allergic to any of them.

Change your child's toothbrush 48 hours after the initiation of the antibiotic treatment to avoid reinfection.

Concerns about latent or delayed complications like rheumatic fever (RF) is why your pediatrician will insist on examining your child and testing for group A streptococcus (GAS). RF is triggered by an immune response against the M protein of GAS which leads to the production of autoreactive antibodies and T cells (T cells are part of the immune system and develop from the stem cells of the bone marrow) that cross-react with the host tissues like heart and/or kidneys. This could lead to post-streptococcal glomerulonephritis. Both conditions could lead to fatal complications. The joints could also be affected.

PANDAS (pediatric autoimmune neuropsychiatric disorders associated with streptococcus infections) is less common, but quite frustrating for parents. Sudden onset of motor tics, obsessive-compulsive disorder (OCD) symptoms, and/or anxiety after GAS infection are the presenting symptoms. If your child suffers from tics, OCD, or anxiety, they may become exacerbated by strep Infection.

In rare cases, your child may become a chronic carrier of GAS when the pharynx is colonized with GAS, but the host is asymptomatic. If your child has recurrent strep infections and still tests positive for the rapid strep antigen test during a period where they are asymptomatic, they are considered chronic carriers. Your pediatrician will help you differentiate true bacterial GAS infections versus asymptomatic chronic carrier and viral pharyngitis.

71. What should I do if my child has ear pain? Is it an ear infection?

Most children have at least one episode of ear pain (otalgia) or an ear infection. Ear infections can present as otitis media (OM), coming from the ancient Greek *oto* for ear and *itis* for inflammation. Acute otitis media (AOM) is one of the most commonly diagnosed conditions in children 1–2 years of age. The ear is formed by an outer ear canal, middle ear, and inner ear. The middle ear is connected with the nasopharynx through a tube called the Eustachian tube.

The reason young children get more frequent infections of the ear is because a child's Eustachian tube is shorter than an adult's and at a different angle in relation to the nasopharynx, which connects the nasal cavity with the soft palate (45 degrees in adults and close to 0 degrees in children, and 35 mm in adults compared to 18 mm in children). Any upper respiratory infection (URI), nasal congestion due to common colds, or bacterial infection in children can complicate AOM. It is important to differentiate AOM from OM with effusion (OME) or fluid buildup behind the tympanic membrane as a result of chronic nasal congestion and inflammation of the sinuses), which rarely requires treatment with antibiotics.

Many children who I follow up with after ER and urgent care visits have been over-diagnosed with AOM and prescribed unnecessary antibiotics. Mild effusion visualized during an otoscopic exam (ear exam) is a result of nasal congestion and mucus build-up in the nasopharynx. Controlling the congestion by irrigating the nasopharynx is the best treatment, and the most efficient.

Because children with both AOM and OME present with pain, analgesics (or pain medications) are prescribed. In the era of infectious disease prevention by vaccine administration, the percentage of bacterial ear infections is lowered to a minimum. As a result, more than 90% of ear pain cases are caused by viruses and require nothing more than supportive treatment and pain management.

Parents sometimes notice symptoms in their infant such as tugging their ears, rubbing their ears on a surface such as a blanket or pillow), fussiness, crying, and fever. If the AOM is diagnosed and proven to be bacterial, it must be treated to avoid complications like hearing loss, suppurative otitis media (an on-going chronic infection of the middle

190

ear) that can cause perforation of the eardrum (tympanic membrane), and mastoiditis (inflammation and pus collection in the mastoid air cells behind the posterior part of the middle ear). Rarely, intracranial infections and abscesses, facial nerve inflammation, and cholesteatoma (an abnormal collection of skin cells deep inside the ear) are diagnosed. If your child develops chronic OM, they may require ear tubes to equalize the pressure in the middle ear, which is a procedure called "myringotomy."

External otitis, also known as "swimmer's ear," causes inflammation of the external ear canal. Swimming, or direct water influx in the ear canal during showering or bathing, increased humidity in tropical climates, foreign bodies like earbuds, hearing devices, or trauma commonly caused by aggressive Q-tip cleansing can all lead to infection of the external canal.

Parents always ask me how to clean the cerumen (earwax) from their children's ears and I love to lecture them on how important earwax is for the ears' protection. It creates an acidic environment that is not favorable for bacterial, viral, or fungal growth.

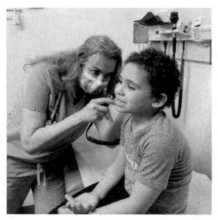

Dr. Daniela Checking for an Ear Infection

I would like to point out one common reason infants tug their ears, and it is a false alarm that brings the children to the doctor's office. When the cerumen builds up, it itches, and the infant becomes fussy and starts touching their ears or rubbing their ears on surfaces like the carpet or a pillow. A gentle cleansing of the ear canals with the protective baby Q-tips after bathing is advisable.

For swimmer's ear prevention, swimmers' ear drops are suggested after water contact because they create an acidic protective environment against fungi and bacteria.

72. How can I tell if my child has pink eye or conjunctivitis?

"Pink eye," "red eye," and "conjunctivitis" are actually all different terminology for the same medical condition. A majority of parents have received a call from the school to pick up their child because of a red eye. Conjunctivitis is the medical diagnosis and it simply means inflammation and redness of the conjunctivae (which is the mucous membrane that covers the front of the eye and inside the eyelids). The conjunctivae is the mucosal lining of the inner part of the upper and inner eyelids, and covers the surface of the eye globe up to the junction of the sclera and cornea. The conjunctiva is generally transparent, but with inflammation, it becomes pink or red, hence they call it "pink eye" or "red eye."

It could be caused by a viral or bacterial infection. If the origin is viral, the redness is mild, the eyes are teary and the secretions are clear or mucousy. Even if there is a crusty discharge, it is whitish or light green in color and occurs mainly in the morning after waking up. In contrast, bacterial conjunctivitis presents with copious mucus and pus. Parents tell me that their child's eyes were "stuck shut" in the morning and the secretions reappeared minutes after wiping the eyelids.

The most common bacterial pathogens in children are *Staphylococcus aureus*, *Haemophilus influenzae*, *Streptococcus pneumoniae*, and *Moraxella catarrhalis*. Antibiotic topical eye drops are used to treat bacterial conjunctivitis.

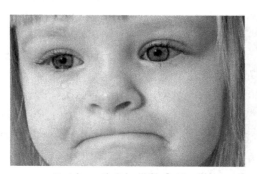

Conjunctivitis/"Pink Eye"

Viral conjunctivitis can present as part of a viral syndrome with associated fever, cough, runny nose, and upper respiratory infection, or it can be an isolated finding affecting only the eye conjunctiva. Regardless of the pathogen, red eye is highly contagious, and hand washing hygiene

194

should be reinforced. Compliance with the treatment is key for prevention of recurrences. Ideally, children may return to school once the discharge has been resolved, but most schools will accept the children 24 hours after the beginning of therapy.

Adenoviruses and their many types have been detected in viral conjunctivitis. Some of the most virulent types—8,19, and 37—have been blamed for severe keratoconjunctivitis, causing inflammation of the cornea, also known as keratitis. The presentation is a, "foreign body-like sensation" which is painful and uncomfortable. It requires urgent medical attention.

Allergic conjunctivitis can be caused by seasonal allergies or animal dander exposure and the itchiness and lack of discharge differentiates it from viral or bacterial pink eye.

Chemical conjunctivitis as a result of toxins like direct perfume or detergent spray in the eye warrants an immediate ophthalmological examination. Any foreign body in the eye is a medical emergency.

73. Does my child have the stomach flu?

"My child has the stomach flu." This is how parents describe gastroenteritis—infection and inflammation of the digestive system—which is another common pediatric diagnosis and condition, caused mainly by viral pathogens. The transmission occurs via oral-fecal direct contact and small epidemic outbursts which are common in daycare centers and schools throughout the year.

Vomiting and/or loose watery stools with abdominal discomfort and bloating, fever, decreased appetite, and/or headache are the presenting symptoms. Hydrating the infant and toddler could be challenging and occasionally requires an ER visit for IV hydration (getting fluids through a thin tube that goes into the vein). The electrolyte balance in infants is very delicate, and pediatricians should spend time educating the parents of a sick child on oral hydration and the worrisome signs of dehydration.

The popular BRAT diet (which is only bananas, rice, applesauce, and toast) is recommended, but its scientific evidence of support is weak. Smaller, frequent meals and fluids are more easily tolerated. Diluted fruit juice, salty crackers, and broths or soups can meet the fluid and salt needs in most cases.

Viral acute gastroenteritis (AGE) is part of common cold viral syndromes and should go away on its own, rarely causing complications. Bacterial AGE has a more acute presentation, and blood is often present in the stool. Traveler's diarrhea is caused by *E. coli*, affecting 30%–40% of the traveling population, thus children become prone to it.

Any blood detected in the stool is a medical emergency, and it is up to the physician to decide what the next steps of treatment will be. Food poisoning, lactose intolerance, food allergies, and certain autoimmune bowel diseases like Crohn's and ulcerative colitis will be considered by your physician.

74. What can I do to help my constipated child?

Constipation is defined by the decreased frequency of bowel movement transition, and the texture of the stool will be hard, "pellet-like" or "ribbon-like." In children, 90% of the constipation diagnoses fall under the category of functional constipation which hardly requires treatment, other than behavioral and/or dietary modifications. The role of the pediatrician is to catch the 5–10% of organic causes. The transition of bowel movements differs throughout childhood development.

Having a normal BM (bowel movement) reflects your child's health. By feeding our "good" and "bad" microbes, we provide food for an estimated 30–100 trillion cells forming our microbiome. The gut is responsible for most of our immune system, and keeping it in check is a great investment. Children are sensitive and emotional creatures, and even a small overreaction of the limbic system (responsible for emotions) will be marked by the gut-brain connection. Do you remember feeling nauseated or like your stomach was tied in a knot? Having the urge to rush to the bathroom? Having a "gut-wrenching" experience? Children go through similar experiences, but because of their young age, they can't explain their symptoms. It is up to the parents and pediatricians to get a detailed history of the symptoms and the circumstances under which abdominal pain and discomfort occur.

The gut has a nervous system called the enteric nervous system, also known as the "second brain." This system functions independently but at the same time is in constant communication with the central nervous system (brain and spinal cord). Having a healthy diet, regular physical activities and exercise, limiting unnecessarily prescribed antibiotics, and controlling stress can help our gut microbiomes to grow in diversity, favoring the good bacteria. Children with previously painful defecation may be afraid to relax their pelvic muscles and will withhold bowel movements. Lack of water and fiber intake, especially for preschoolers and kindergarteners who are still working on their independence skills, is another common reason for constipation.

My favorite tip for constipated children and their parents is to offer lots of fruits that start with the letter "P" to help your child poop:

- Pears
- Prunes
- Papaya
- Pineapple
- Pumpkin
- Peaches

In newborns and infants, changes of formula and taking iron supplements haven't shown strong evidence to be related to hard stool. I always discourage my parents from chaotically changing baby formulas in the hopes this will improve the frequency and texture of the stool. My approach is to work with the child, providing cognitive behavioral therapy (CBT) and progressive muscle relaxation (PMR) with the help of psychologists, behavioral and developmental specialists, and GI doctors.

If there are any red flags like weight loss, bloody stool, painful bowel evacuation, and abnormal blood work on labs, I work in close contact with the gastroenterologist to finalize the diagnosis and provide treatment. Love your fruits and veggies, have family meals, purchase healthy groceries, and cook with your children.

75. Does my child have a cold or bronchiolitis? What can I do to help?

Bronchiolitis is a diagnosis used to describe the inflammation of the lower respiratory airways in children 0–2 years of age. Common cold viruses are prevalent during the cool months of the year (autumn to spring), and are the main pathogens behind the disease. It is a demanding task to take care of a sick child, but with newborns, infants, and toddlers, it is even more taxing. They may have difficulties feeding and latching due to nasal congestion. Plus, they act fussier and weaker which leads to decreased appetite, all of which are symptoms that seem worrisome to parents.

As a pediatrician with over 20 years of experience, I have developed skills to examine the behavior and reaction of the child during physical examination. It is so important to be able to keep the child calm by distracting them to examine the lungs, throat, and ears.

My medical students are well-taught on how to differentiate a severely ill child from a stable and comfortable child with mild symptoms of a common cold. Bronchiolitis is different from an upper respiratory infection (URI), which is limited to the upper airways. Bronchiolitis or inflammation of the bronchioles (the small airways in the lower respiratory tract) is preceded by upper respiratory infection. It usually peaks on day 2–3 and lasts for about 10–14 days on average. By day 21, 90% of children will have typically recovered, and the cough will be resolved without any treatment.

Hydration and keeping the nasal airways open are helpful treatments for the symptoms. Inhaled hypertonic saline is seldomly needed, and yet it is sometimes used in an ER setting. It is important to differentiate between bronchiolitis—which causes bronchospasm or wheezing—from an asthma attack because it is a viral illness.

Your pediatrician will make the final diagnosis, but the treatment may be the same. All cases and children are treated based on their previous medical history and current clinical presentation. A cough, runny nose, and fever are the most common symptoms. When the child flares their nostrils, it means they are having trouble breathing and/or the oxygen saturation is low. The child is in distress, so hospital admission may be advised for further treatment and observation of your child.

CHAPTER SIX: SLEEP (PAST A YEAR OLD)

Dr. Shellie's Mom Memories of Her Children's Sleep

The other day, I joked with a medical professional who was seeing my teenager that I needed to talk about "children sleeping" in this book and that I shouldn't be the one to write this because, "at 14 years old, he still doesn't sleep through the night!" All kidding aside, when it comes to sleep and children, it can be very difficult to master a sleep schedule. Sometimes children (and their loving caretakers) are not naturally on a typical circadian rhythm which is the process that regulates the sleep-wake schedule that is considered to be normal.

I can only stress that, for young children, creating and sticking to a nighttime routine can be very beneficial. We did have a routine when they were young that included tooth brushing, baths, quiet soothing music, and diffusing calming essential oils, and I always read a book or two to my kiddos once they were snuggled into their cribs or beds. Create a pattern that you can follow at night that will soothe them and let their brains know that it is in fact time to sleep.

Read on to learn how Dr. Daniela responds to questions from her patient's parents about getting proper rest. Best wishes for a peaceful night's sleep for you and your child.

Dr. Daniela's Pediatric Prescription for Children's Sleep

76. How many hours should my child sleep?

Sleep, like water and food, is essential for human survival. Sleep is the time our bodily functions slow down and "recharge," the subconsciousness is tested, and the brain registers it as a dream. Even the embryo (your baby in utero) follows the circadian rhythms and the sleep patterns of the mother.

Sleep Requirements by Age

Infants, 4–12 months of age: 12–16 hours (including naps)

Toddlers, 1–2-year-old children: 11–14 hours (including naps)

3–5-year-old children: 10–13 hours (including naps)

6–12-year-old children: 9–12 hours

Teens, 13–18-year-old children: 8–10 hours

These recommendations are made by the American Academy of Sleep Medicine and endorsed by the AAP. Every annual exam of mine includes a question about sleep and its characteristics. It is so important for a pediatrician to ask specific questions about bedtime issues, like:

- "Does your child have a bedtime routine?"
- "Is your infant able to soothe themselves and go back to sleep in the middle of the night after awakening?"
- "How interrupted is their sleep at night?"
- "Are there unusual behaviors during sleep, like night terrors, nightmares, sleepwalking, and/or abnormal movements?"
- "Does your child demand co-sleeping and move to your bed in the middle of the night?"
- "Is your child a mouth breather or do they snore at night?"

Once I take a detailed history of the sleep disturbances, I like to also get familiar with the family dynamics, day or night shifts of parents' work schedules, the schedules of other siblings, dinner times, and details about the sleeping environment. The environment can provide comfort in sleep, but at the same time disrupt sleep patterns. Every case and family situation is different, and I address this issue with counseling on a weekly and monthly basis.

77. How can I get my child to go to sleep on time when they resist it?

Bedtime routines are important, but they are often overlooked by parents. We get caught up in our busy lives and, many times, are forced to simply let the children entertain themselves with screen time till they fall asleep.

Living in New York, I have learned that most of my parents are maintaining two jobs, working day and night shifts, and hardly have energy to spend time with their children at night. Infants are fed and put to sleep, but toddlers and preschool children are often left alone in their rooms to play with their older siblings till they fall asleep.

Less attention is paid to books and quiet evening routines. Audiobooks are the preferred way of reading and sadly this is done by technology, not the parents. The human connection is partially lost in these modern times, but how can we reinforce and rebuild human family interactions and deepen the connection? It is a complex topic, as family dynamics could vary from a struggling single mother with financial insecurities to a mom with an abusive partner in the home.

In a healthy family environment, it is easy to advise the parents to set up daily routines like early dinner, walking the dog, and a warm bath, followed by teeth brushing, and reading time with mom, dad, or an older sibling. All parents want the best for their children. If the children are opposed to sleep, one does not have to give up easily; I encourage them to build healthy habits, even if it takes some positive reward and reinforcement. Getting to know the families and the parents' relationship helps me evaluate the situation and come up with a plan. In some cases, I would reach out to a psychologist, a neurodevelopmental specialist, and a sleep therapist. Children with ADHD, ASD, developmental delays, and special needs often present with sleep disturbances and struggle with going to bed on time.

78. How can I stop my child from waking up in the middle of the night and coming to sleep in our bed?

Co-sleeping with your newborn and its risks for suffocation and SIDS were discussed earlier in the book. Under no circumstances would I accept co-sleeping with a newborn. Toddlers and preschoolers, however, tend to wake up in the middle of the night and snuggle in their parent's bed. This is the age they start exploring the world, experiencing emotions, meeting new friends, learning how to socialize, and attending school. Their sleep is not always deep and uninterrupted. They need reassurance and their fears are real, but it is up to us, the grownups, to determine how to handle it all, and help them overcome their fears.

It takes patience and consistency to teach your child how to remain calm and comfortable in their own bedroom. Once you allow them to invade your bed, they get confused, and it will take longer to break this habit.

Make sure their room is comfortable and there is nothing in it that frightens them. Spend time with your child in their room for pleasant activities. If they walk into your room, walk them back and sit on their bed, or wait behind the door until they fall asleep again. For older kids, you may encourage them to fall asleep with their favorite toy and keep a night light on.

79. What should I do if my child wakes up in the middle of the night and wants to play until early morning?

This is another scenario I continue to hear from my parents. Usually around the ages of 2–4 years, children wake up soon after midnight and insist on playing with toys and being with their parents until they get exhausted and pass out. The first questions I ask in cases like this are, "How did they spend their day? Did they nap more than usual?

Was there any unusual excitement? Are there any stress factors or drastic changes in their routines?" If we can't connect those answers to the cause, then I run a detailed questionnaire and look for other possible underlying diseases.

Sometimes the circadian rhythm of your child is a bit off, and even if you do your best, they can have sleep disturbances and unexplained awakenings in the middle of the night. I remember many nights of play with my daughter who refused to sleep between 2 a.m. and 5 a.m. We used to play imaginary games and were chasing the cats in the house until early morning.

Sleep disturbances are very commonly associated with hyperactivity (as a family trait, not necessarily a full-blown disease), developmental delays, and autism spectrum disorder (ASD). Rarely, medications are needed, but in cases where all other options have been explored, melatonin could be used, usually after psychiatric and neuropsychological evaluation.

80. Why does my child wake up screaming in the middle of the night?

Night terrors occur in the middle of the night, usually 2–4 hours after falling asleep. Children wake up and start screaming, jumping out of their bed, and running away from something that is scary to them. During a night terror, you won't be able to calm your child even if you try. Their hearts are racing. They are flushed and sweaty. The episodes last about 10–20 minutes and can happen 2 to 3 times per week. All you have to do as a parent is to assure the safety of your child until they fall back to sleep.

Sometimes children have the same nightmare over and over. In my son's recurring dream, it was based on his real-life experiences. When he was 9 years old, his tennis coach at the time came up with a game where Daniel had to hit 1,000 balls in a row on the tennis court without a mistake. It took Daniel about three months until he successfully made all those 1,000 balls in a row. During this time, he would scream in his sleep. He would physically "hit" groundstrokes while counting out loud "966, 967, 968…" He had no recollection of this event in the morning. I secretly videotaped him, and we would laugh out loud together the next day watching the video.

Night terrors occur with no reason, or during an illness accompanied by a fever, and/or sleep deprivation. Stick to your healthy bedtime routines and make sure your child gets enough sleep. Night terrors are associated with non-rapid eye movement (NREM). Sleep studies using an electroencephalogram (EEG) to record brain activity may show high-amplitude rhythmic delta and theta activity (brain wave activity). There is a strong genetic predisposition for night terrors, so if someone in your family has experienced night terrors, it is quite possible that your child's DNA is wired in the same way.

Nightmares on the other hand are scary dreams occurring during REM sleep in the final stage of sleep, usually in the early morning hours just before waking up. Scary movies or books, unpleasant or terrifying day experiences, and anxiety can all cause nightmares. Older kids may recall some of their dreams. Setting up calm bedtime routines and playing soothing music could be helpful.

81. How can we stop my child from sleepwalking?

Sleepwalking is another sleep disruption during non-rapid eye movement (NREM) sleep. It is more common in children older than 7–12 years of age but could be seen in preschoolers, even though it is rare. The child will wake up quietly, sitting on the edge of the bed, then get off the bed, and walk around in the room or house. A lot of times, this behavior is left unnoticed if constrained to the child's room.

I was "lucky enough" to watch my daughter Stefani sleepwalk until she was 12 years old, because she had the habit of running to my room in the middle of the night to cuddle with me. She would get up in the middle of the night and start walking in the room, open the door, and take the stairs down to the living room. It is amazing how accurately they can self-orient in the darkness and how difficult it is to wake them up during their sleepwalk. You can redirect them, guide them, and help them go back to their bedroom and bed.

Rarely do those who sleepwalk engage in dangerous behaviors and hurt themselves. The condition is typically outgrown, but if persistent and puts the child in danger, (like for example leaving the house in cold weather) a sleep therapist, neurologist, and psychiatrist must counsel the child.

82. What should I do if my child snores and stops breathing in the middle of the night?

Some of the causes of snoring at night include chronic rhinitis, sinusitis, enlarged tonsils or adenoids, and frequent tonsil infections. Infants and toddlers suffering from frequent common colds and bronchiolitis have congested noses and are commonly labeled as "mouth breathers." If your child stops breathing for a few seconds, you must inform your pediatrician because this could be part of a diagnosis called obstructive sleep apnea (OSA). OSA is a worrisome diagnosis that needs to be addressed and treated immediately. I always ask my parents to provide me with a video recording of their child's snoring to guide me through the diagnostic process.

A healthy child falls asleep quickly and has quiet breathing. With OSA, there is an increased resistance in the upper airways during sleep, which leads to increased work to breathe with snoring resulting in sleep disruption. OSA is caused by the complete or partial collapse of one or more of the extrathoracic (the structures supporting the pharynx and lungs) segments of the airways.

Some causes could be genetic, for example: when the babies are born with anatomically small airways, have genetic diseases with anatomical abnormalities like a small chin or mandible, are hypoplastic (smaller face), or have macroglossia (enlarged tongue). Other non-genetic causes are asthma, allergic rhinitis, sinusitis, obesity, adenotonsillar hypertrophy, or neuromuscular diseases like cerebral palsy.

Regardless of the underlying condition, OSA will require sleep apnea studies where your child will be expected to spend a night in the hospital as they monitor their breathing and oxygen delivered to the tissues. OSA leads to hypoventilation or decreased

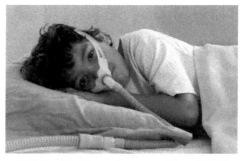

Child with Sleep Apnea with a CPAP Machine

oxygen delivered to the main vital organs like the brain, heart, and lungs. As a result, your child can present with nightmares, bed wetting, irritability, day sleepiness, fatigue, morning headaches, lack of concentration, and a short attention span. Once the diagnosis is confirmed, your doctor will refer you to an ENT specialist where a plan of treatment will be made.

I recall the ENT specialist who operated on my son when he was 2 years of age. His words were, "Don't beat yourself up. It's just bad luck." Dr. Vikash Modi, a pediatric ENT specialist affiliated with Cornell Hospital meant that the anatomical structure of the sinuses and the nasopharyngeal airways were not favorable enough and were causing sinus infections triggered by common colds. Daniel suffered from recurrent sinusitis requiring monthly antibiotics, one CT scan of the brain, two hospital admissions, and countless sleepless nights with loud snoring, which used to terrify me. Eventually, his adenoids were removed and his breathing and sleep became comfortable. Being in close contact with your pediatrician and the ENT specialist will help in the diagnostic process and the final decision for what would be best for your child, either ear tubes, removal of the adenoids and tonsils, or all of the above.

83. Why does my baby shake during sleep, and why do their muscles twitch?

Upon falling asleep, our body is preparing for the transition from awakening to falling asleep. It is a smooth transition involving all of our organs, but the brain is the conductor of the orchestra, metaphorically speaking. Brief and sudden muscle jerking movements are spontaneous and often called "sleep starts" or "hypnic jerks." These are benign muscle movements seen during drifting off to sleep and accompanied by a dream-like feeling or flashing sensations.

Parents will often video record and share their concerns with the pediatrician. Stereotyped, brief movements or repetitive jerks of the extremities and the trunk during sleep in infants less than 6 months of age are often seen in the recordings.

Important questions for the pediatrician to ask are:

- Timing related to sleep onset.
- Duration and frequency of the events.
- Description and nature of the movements—for instance, whether they occur randomly any time during a 24-hour period or are stereotyped, which means they occur in a particular pattern, such as only during the day, only at night, or with certain activities.
- Localization and distribution—focal (only one part of the body involved) or generalized (the whole body and all extremities are involved).

- Alertness and consciousness during the events.

These will help the doctor decide if the nature of the movement is benign and if only reassurance and observation are needed. A neurologist must be involved to differentiate epileptic movements or seizures, restless leg syndrome, sleep-related leg cramping, or rhythmic movement disorder.

Pay attention to all the details and questions that your doctor will expect you to answer, and video the sleep events before your doctor's visit to help your pediatrician make the right diagnosis.

84. Can I give melatonin to my child to help them fall asleep?

Childhood insomnia or sleep disturbances can cause significant distress for the whole family. Parasomnia is a sleep disorder that can include symptoms such as talking in your sleep and having abnormal movements while sleeping. Bedtime resistance, difficulties initiating sleep, and frequent night awakenings due to parasomnias are perhaps some of the most commonly asked questions during a well child visit during the ages of 1 to 5 years. Like most of my colleagues and fellow pediatricians, I recommend behavioral modifications first. Spending an ample amount of time with the family and asking them to fill out a sleep questionnaire before the visit helps provide the answers. If the child has neurological and/or psychiatric underlying disease or physical developmental delays sleep medication could be considered if the behavioral modifications fail.

Melatonin is a hormone secreted by the pineal gland of the brain in response to decreased light, and using it as a medication is usually considered for children with ADHD or ASD (autism spectrum disorder) because they often have delayed onset of sleep and demonstrate sleep resistance. The medication starts acting in approximately 60 minutes after administration. Even though melatonin is an over-the-counter medication, I strongly advise against using it without consulting your pediatrician first. There are other pharmacological options available, such as antihistamine medications, benzodiazepines, and antidepressants; if needed, your pediatrician or neurologist may recommend or prescribe them.

CHAPTER SEVEN: EATING (BEYOND 1 YEAR OLD)

Dr. Shellie's Mom Memories of Her Children Eating

Eating together as a family can be such a beautiful way to bond. Meal times spent together discussing the day's events and trying new foods can make for wonderful memories. With my two children, they have very different eating routines. Alyssa has always loved to eat a variety of foods, try new dishes, and even learned to use chopsticks before she used a fork. Jacob, on the other hand, doesn't deviate from his menu very much, and that could have something to do with his ASD. Because he's on the spectrum, he struggles in restaurants with hearing other people chewing (his hearing is very sensitive), and he doesn't like to veer off from what he typically eats—both in food choices and in the way it is prepared. He likes his routine.

This chapter addresses everything from underweight/overweight children and their needs to how to deal with dietary concerns. I encourage you to make a healthy snack for you and your child and then gobble up this chapter on eating!

Dr. Daniela's Pediatric Prescription for Children's Eating

85. We are a vegan family. What will happen to my child if we don't serve meat at our home?

No one can argue the fact that nutrition is the most important environmental factor for lifelong health and longevity. Anti-aging and health are topics that have gained popularity in the last decade. From the second we are born, we impact our longevity and health. From being delivered vaginally and exposed to the mother's vaginal microbiome, to breastfeeding and introduction to non-processed and clean meals in the first two years of life, to growing up as an adolescent and becoming an independent young adult making healthy meal choices, all these factors are intertwined.

The moment one is born, one is at risk. Within an hour of your baby's first breath and cry they will be offered mom's breast milk. It is up to the parents to make the decision regarding how to feed their newborn. Fortunately, maternal instincts are very strong and the majority of my mothers are willing to breastfeed if they can, for as long as they can.

Every culture comes with its traditions and cuisine. I have learned to respect and accept different cuisines and to be flexible and appreciative of parents' beliefs. Vegan parents are often concerned about the lack of animal products in their diets and if this will have a negative effect on the newborn's growth.

The diet of the mother won't affect the quality of the breast milk. Regardless of your dietary restrictions, the baby will be getting all the benefits from breast milk. Its composition and nutritional value will be the same. The ability of a mother to breastfeed and the amount of milk depends on the frequency and amount sucked out of the breast by their newborn. This has been shown in multiple research studies on twins and triplets.

During the lactation period, every mom has increased caloric and nutritional needs. In cases of severely restricted diets and because of the fact that all fat- and water-soluble vitamins are transmitted through breast milk, every mother must supplement those high demands. A balanced and clean diet is ideal for every mother's health, but without animal products in your diet, it can be hard to get the right nutrients. A nursing mother who eats a vegan diet should consider prenatal vitamins, as well as vitamin B12 supplementation. Bone mineralization is diminished during pregnancy and lactation, so vitamin D and calcium, which are included in the prenatal vitamins, are important to maintaining bone mass. I support parents either way, but bear in mind that you might be more prone to nutrient deficiencies that can impact your health.

86. Is my child overweight? Why does my child obsess about food?

The obesity epidemic started in the late 1980s in the United States, but it is now an international and global problem. In children, we use different criteria to classify "obesity."

Body Mass Index (BMI) which measures body fat based on weight and height in adult men and women has normal ranges between 18.5 and 24.9. In children, we use the same BMI but instead of metric units, we base it on the percentile for age. Anything from the 5th to 85th percentile is considered normal, 85th to 95th percentile overweight, and above 95th percentile obese. Ask your pediatrician to always provide you with the growth chart for your child.

Obesity and children being overweight is multifactorial. In rare cases there is a genetic, autoimmune, or metabolic disease causing excess weight gain. Being sensitive and understanding during the parent's and patient's interview is important. A judgmental attitude can cause trauma and lead to self-destructive behaviors and eating disorders later on in life.

Understanding the core problem like family habits and the child's daily routine by obtaining a diet diary and getting an idea of the child's daily life can determine the approach towards nutrition and treatment. Obesity at an early age is a risk factor for metabolic syndrome, diabetes, heart disease, and so many comorbidities that will require chronic therapy and care in the long term.

The main focus should be on communicating and staying in touch with the parents to make behavioral changes and set realistic goals. A frequent question I get from my parents is, "How much weight does my child need to lose?" The approach for weight loss in children is different, as maintaining the weight and reaching

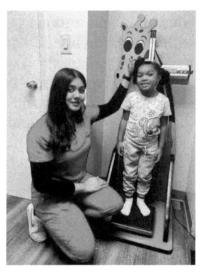

Child at Dr. Daniela's Office on a Scale

healthy proportions for the child's weight compared to their height is the goal. Growing children require specific daily caloric needs. A nutritionist will follow up on progress of weight changes monthly and work closely with the family members and caretakers.

I have seen the most success from group therapy and close up counseling with me in person or through telehealth visits. The main obstacles are educating and influencing the parents, working with the children, and creating a plan. Adopting a new lifestyle is a slow and lengthy process that, sadly, frequently fails. According to recent (2021) statistics from the World Health Organization, an estimated 38 million children worldwide under the age of 5 are obese. Putting these numbers together with the 3.1 million children dying annually from starvation is a disturbing fact.

87. How can I expand my baby's food selections? Why does my baby only eat soft foods?

Most babies are ready to start the introduction of solids around 6 months of age, and the AAP recommends starting solid foods at 4–6 months of age. To be ready to eat solid food, the baby must be at a certain level of physical development for the food to be processed properly. Chewing solid food requires perfect coordination between smashing up food in the mouth to form a bolus and then pushing that food into and down the esophagus (feeding tube). Once the food is in the esophagus, small contractions known as peristalsis push the food down to the lower sphincter of the esophagus and into the stomach.

Even though pediatricians recommend starting solids at 4–6 months, nothing is written in stone. There are many valid reasons your infant may refuse solids, including not liking the texture or taste of the food, fighting the spoon in the mouth because they recognize it as a foreign object, being forced or fed too quickly without allowing time to chew, being fed while not hungry, and being offered food that is not pureed and cooked properly.

Refusing certain textures of food may be part of a sensory integration disorder, where the brain overreacts and does not accept certain textures or tastes. Regardless of the reasons, when parents come to me, all they say is, "My child is such a picky eater. I don't know what to do." In my practice, I have a questionnaire that helps me recognize the reasons behind the picky baby/toddler when it comes to eating.

Picky Eater Questionnaire

- How do you know that your child is hungry?
- How do you know your child is not hungry?
- What is the feeding environment?
- How do you prepare the baby's food?
- Does the family have some religious or cultural beliefs about restricting certain foods?
- How much breastmilk/formula and/or juice do you offer to your child in a 24-hour period?
- Is the child pushing the food, spitting it out, or gagging once you introduce the food and bring it to their mouth?
- Is your child vomiting soon after the feedings?
- Is your child teething?
- Does your child have a common cold?

- Is your child having normal bowel movements?
- Are there any stress factors or recent changes in the family dynamics?
- Are both parents healthy? Is there any domestic violence or chronic illness?

The answers to these questions provide clues that will lead me to understand how best to approach each and every unique case. In New York, I have had the pleasure to work with occupational therapists (OTs) who have provided excellent feeding therapy care. When it comes to diet, feeding, and growth development, the most successful approach is providing home care OT professionals or home care nurses who can study the family environment, spend time with the caregivers, and get to know and work with the child individually.

In the short 15–30 min of an annual examination in the office, I can only reassure the parents about the growth of their child. If there is a growth developmental delay based on the growth curves and/or comorbidities which contribute to poor growth, the approach is completely different, and further investigations are needed.

88. What should I pack for my child's school lunch?

Being a mother of two, I often recall the chaotic school day mornings. Days began with waking up the kids, dressing them up, prepping breakfast, assisting with brushing their teeth followed by packing lunch boxes, and driving them to school. It seems like an impossible task to complete. Imagine that you have to do this every single day for many years to come. This is the morning of almost every parent, and it is often followed by going to work where they have to be at their best.

Luckily for me, I had help from my mother who is still a devoted and loving grandmother. She makes sure my kids and I have freshly cooked meals that are well-balanced with clean, non-processed foods and snacks. My son is a nationally ranked tennis player who competes at the international level, and as you would imagine, there are many nutritional requirements for a growing male teenager who spends three hours on the tennis court practicing daily!

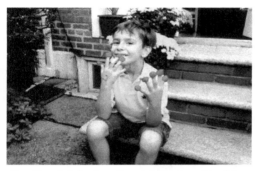

Dr. Daniela's Son Daniel Eating Healthy Berries

Some children have a natural interest in preparing their own lunch, but others don't. Lunch food in U.S. schools is typically not well-balanced and not always tasty. Overwhelming amounts of carbs and fattening fast food-style choices are offered. In contrast, I will never forget the delicious, quality meals I used to have in my school growing up in Bulgaria. It would be unfair to compare a country like Bulgaria, with a population of only 7 million, to the United States, with a population of 330 million (with more than

50 million school-aged children).[2] It is not easy to provide, prepare, and offer fresh foods for such an enormous population.

I personally encourage my parents to learn how to prepare lunch boxes for their kids and involve them in the process. Shopping together, becoming an active participant, and cooking is a shared healthy hobby.

My ideal lunch box meal ideas, depending on the culture and food preferences, would be:

- Salad, a bowl of soup and rice or potatoes with a piece of meat or fish. Desert would be either a fruit or homemade cookie.
- Pasta with fresh tomato sauce with some protein in the form of lean meats, fish, or ground beef; mushrooms; olives; and cheese is a cooked lunch that could be reheated.

---

[2] https://www.worldometers.info/world-population/population-by-country

- A sandwich made out of whole-grain bread with lettuce, tomatoes, sliced cheese, and smoked salmon is another favorite.

Being organized is very important when you have children in the house. Shopping during the weekend and cooking for a few days in advance provides pre-prepped food to stay on track. Freezing the soups and fruit purees can certainly help. Every parent wants to raise a healthy child. The job of the pediatrician is to keep reinforcing and reminding them that the best investment in the health of their children is with healthy food choices.

CHAPTER EIGHT: SPECIAL NEEDS AND CHRONIC HEALTH CONDITIONS

Dr. Shellie's Mom Memories of Special Needs and Chronic Health Conditions

As I explained earlier, I spent much of my working life dedicated to people with special needs, and I have a son who has been diagnosed with ASD and ADHD. I have had amazing students who have been in almost all areas of special education including students who were Deaf and grew up to live great lives within the Deaf community and culture.

The technology available now for children who are differently-abled can open up so many new strategies and opportunities for learning. There are great educational techniques to help your child to learn and interact. Plus, many coping skills can be taught that will help bridge the gap for them physically, emotionally, behaviorally, or academically.

I want you to know as a parent that whatever your child's needs are, you will find ways to meet them. I would urge you to "meet your child where they are" by finding out who your child is beyond their special needs. While you need to know medically and educationally what they need for their emotional, physical, and mental health—it is also important to get to know their abilities, their strengths, and what they like. Every child is unique, and inside all children is something special. They can learn and live their best quality of life when you do your research about their needs, differentiate to create a plan that will help them, and approach parenting with love.

If your child is diagnosed with a special need ranging from a chronic health condition such as cystic fibrosis to a neurodivergence such as autism spectrum disorder (ASD), it will be important for you to read Dr. Daniela's responses to these important parent questions. Also, we live

242

in a world filled with differently-abled children and it's important that we have an understanding of their needs and how we can support each other.

Dr. Daniela's Pediatric Prescription for Children with Special Needs and Chronic Health Conditions

89. Why does my child have asthma? What is causing the asthma, and is it for life?

Asthma is one of the most commonly diagnosed chronic diseases in pediatrics, both in the emergency room and in the outpatient clinical settings. I am so incredibly pleased and proud of the progress made in the treatment of asthma over the last two decades. I was raised in the Balkans, on a semi-island where the label "asthma" sounded like a death sentence. Families would relocate in the mountainous areas away from the heavily polluted urban cities.

As a medical student, I hardly remember examining one or two children with wheezes and have never seen even one asthma exacerbation; hence, during my schooling I didn't learn how to manage and treat it, not to mention that, in the late 1980s, there were limited treatment options in my country. The best choice was the fresh purified mountain air scented with evergreens and pine trees.

As a pediatric resident at Mount Sinai, I was taught that asthma is the most common chronic respiratory illness in children. In less than two decades, I have witnessed such success in the care of my little happy and not-so-happy "wheezers."

Wheezing is the medical term for what parents described as, "my child is making a whistling sound when breathing." Asthma is a chronic disease that has three components: airflow obstruction, bronchial hyper-responsiveness, and inflammatory reaction. Triggers can be the climate, cold weather, exercise, seasonal changes, viral illnesses, inhaled chemicals, food allergens, animal allergens like cat or dog dander, cockroaches, rodents, and dust mites.

It could be challenging to diagnose a child with asthma, especially under the age of 5 when common colds are indeed so common that a child attending school will catch 8 to 10 of them in a year. Cough, nasal congestion, shortness of breath, and wheezing with occasional chest tightness are the symptoms presented in asthma. They frequently overlap the symptoms of common cold illnesses.

I like to follow up with all children who present with wheezing every 3 months even if they haven't had any sickness in between. By reviewing the chronicity and severity of their symptoms, it helps me come out with an asthma action plan based on their classification: mild, moderate, moderate persistent, or severe. Avoiding the triggers if possible is the best initial approach.

When evaluating for asthma, your doctor should ask:

- Is your child coughing more in school and at home compared to when they are outdoors? (This could be a dust mite clue).
- Is your child reacting to humid and hot versus cold weather?

- Is your child exposed to second-hand smoke?
- Do you have rodents or cockroaches in the house?
- Does your child cough after exercise or when running around in the house (exercise-induced asthma causes shortness of breath and wheezing 10–15 minutes after the end of exercise)?
- Does your child end up with a "whistling cough" and bronchospasm (wheezing) every time they catch a viral respiratory infection?

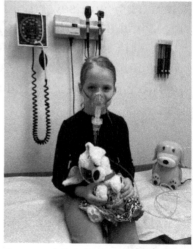

Asking about the family history of asthma is also important to determine the risk of the child getting the disease. Known food allergies, a

Dr. Daniela's Office, Child with Asthma with Nebulizer

history of eczema or atopic dermatitis, and allergic rhinitis, can all lead to the diagnosis of asthma. Being in close contact with your pediatrician and compliance with the medications will determine the outcome of your asthma presentation and exacerbations.

Fortunately, most bronchospastic airway diseases that we label as being "asthma" before the age of 5 are outgrown. If the exacerbations persist beyond the age of 5 and are recurrent, then asthma is likely to remain a chronic condition.

90. Why does my child suffer from chronic eczema? How can I help their skin heal?

"Atopic dermatitis" is the diagnosis your pediatrician will give for eczema. Eczema is a chronic inflammation of the skin that causes dryness and itchiness, and presents with scaly and red patches of the skin with specific distribution patterns based on age. With a family history of atopic dermatitis, asthma, and/or allergic rhinitis, the child can be at increased risk for eczema. If one parent is affected by the above "triad" of medical conditions, the evidence shows that the child would have a two- to threefold higher chance of developing atopic dermatitis; if two of the parents are affected, the chances will increase to three or four times.

You can imagine the disappointment of my new parents when they have to deal with skin conditions in general, but especially eczema, which affects a large surface of the body's skin and does not spare the face.

There are a few theories about atopic dermatitis. The first is that it is generally hereditary, and the second is that it is caused by dysregulation of the gene for filaggrin, which is also genetically inherited and causes disruption of the skin barrier capability for water retention and environmental protection. The "hygiene hypothesis" also supports the fact that less interaction with endotoxins (a toxin inside the bacterial cell released during the cell disintegration), lack of early daycare attendance, living in urban areas (versus rural with exposure to farms and animals), and not being raised with a pet increases the risks for atopy, including skin conditions like atopic dermatitis.

Food allergens caused by genetic and environmen tal factors can worsen the condition of atopic dermatitis,

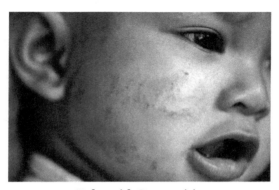

Baby with Dermatitis

but are seldomly the main cause for it. The highest prevalence of eczema is in the first 2 years of life, but in rare cases, it can last longer and even into adulthood.

You can manage atopic dermatitis by eliminating triggers, keeping the skin moist, applying emollients right after showering and bathing, controlling the inflammation during flare-ups, and treating the infection when the skin microbiome is imbalanced because of bacterial overgrowth.

Topical steroids, bleach baths, immunomodulator topical drugs (regulating the local immune response of the skin), and antibiotics as necessary are all possible ways of controlling and treating this skin condition. If allergy skin testing is needed, your pediatrician will refer you to an allergist and immunologist, and a second opinion from a dermatologist may be considered.

91. Does my child have an immune deficiency if they get sick often?

Isn't this the epic question of every parent with a toddler who attends daycare? I like to tell my parents that if we want to coexist with nature and live on planet earth we have to learn how to live together. Because the genomes of humans differ from the ones of other living organisms, we need to get to know each other, and the only way to do this is through meeting each other. As a pediatrician, it is my job to differentiate between a child with a healthy immune system and one with an immune deficiency. Typically, a child with a "normal"

252

immune system will get an average of 8 to 10 common cold infections a year and successfully recover.

I have been the luckiest pediatrician, because most of my patients and the children I've followed in outpatient clinics have been healthy and able to bounce back from common illnesses. Several studies show that the most predictive factor for primary immunodeficiency (PID) is family history. The overall incidence of PID is 1 in 10,000 and is greater in boys than in girls (Varadhi, et al., 2013). Underlying chronic diseases, prematurity, and previous surgical procedures can result in secondary immunodeficiencies (Reda, et al., 2013).

Here are some signs that a child may have PID:

- Four or more new ear infections within one year.
- Two or more serious sinus infections in one year.
- Poor response to antibiotics.
- Two or more pneumonias in one year.

- Failure of an infant to gain weight or grow normally.
- Recurrent, deep skin or organ abscesses.
- Persistent thrush in mouth or fungal infection on skin.
- Need for intravenous antibiotics to clear infections.
- Two or more deep-seated infections, including septicemia (blood infection leading to toxic shock).
- A family history of PI.

The infection history and its duration, frequency, and treatment response, together with the growth development will be used by your doctor to decide if further investigation, genetic and immunologic studies, or referrals to an immunologist are needed.

Immunodeficiencies are extremely rare, so there is no need to panic. However, following up with your pediatrician is advisable.

92. Do you recommend a special diet for children on the autism spectrum? What extracurricular activities and academic pursuits supports would be best for them? How can I best help my child on the spectrum?

Having a child who has been diagnosed per the Diagnostic and Statistical Manual (DSM) as on the autism spectrum, means that they have autism spectrum disorder (ASD). This is an important diagnosis, and the sooner it is made, the better the outcome. There are so many different forms of ASD, and every child with this diagnosis will require an individualized approach and a team of doctors (neurodevelopmental pediatrician, child psychiatrist, child neurologist, and child neuropsychologist) with the active participation of parents and teachers.

Parents have been challenging me through the years with questions that I was not always ready or able to answer like, "Is there a special diet for children on the autism spectrum?" Some parents start restricting their children from important macro and micronutrients without any scientific evidence. The most common diet that parents adopt for their children on the spectrum is gluten-free, lactose-free, and plant-based. Lactose and gluten are well-known inflammatory agents, but sadly, there is no proof that avoiding them helps children on the autism spectrum in any positive way. What I personally advise my parents about diet is to provide a variety of fresh and non-processed foods under the guidance of a nutritionist.

In terms of activities, there are certain sports that have been shown in research studies to improve the way children on the autism spectrum process their emotions and feelings, and they also change how they view their environment. For example, horseback riding can help stimulate the senses like smell, touch, and hearing, as well as help their coordination and balance. Learning how to control the horse by giving commands using their bodies without the need to talk builds up confidence and skills that help them function better in social situations where communication is needed.

There is research based-evidence for the benefits of hippotherapy (therapeutic horseback riding). In a randomized trial that compared 10 weeks of therapeutic horseback riding with 10 weeks of barn activity not

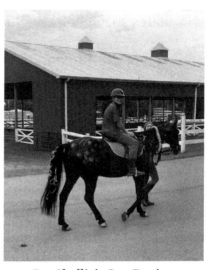

Dr. Shellie's Son During Horseback Therapy

involving horses in 116 children with ASD, hippotherapy appeared to improve the irritability and hyperactivity after approximately 5 weeks. Hippotherapy also improved social cognition and social communication as assessed by parents' reports. Attention span, social motivation, and distractibility were all improved (Bass & Llabre, 2009). Even though hippotherapy is not largely included in the routine care of children with ASD, it is definitely something I recommend.

Having a pet also reduces social stress and stimulates social behaviors in children with ASD.

For highly functioning children with ASD, all sports are beneficial, but slow exposure starting with individual sports is advisable. The goal is to work on their motor skills and take advantage of the physical activities by simultaneously improving their social interactions and building confidence and self-esteem.

Tennis is a sport that helps with hand-eye coordination and movement. Individual sports help children deal with the anxiety of engaging in conversations and communication with potential team players. Tennis, golf, swimming, skiing, gymnastics, chess, and martial arts are all great choices. It is always worth exposing a child with ASD to team sports as long as they like it, and it is not overwhelmingly and socially frustrating. Every child should be approached individually.

Sadly, most children with ASD end up with one or more additional diagnoses like oppositional defiant, combative, and ADHD. There might be co-existing disorders that require medical attention and treatment. Helping the children become more independent and more confident in their daily social interactions is a main goal of every parent and pediatrician when it comes to children who are on the spectrum.

93. When should children's vision and hearing tests be performed? Is it done in the office, or do I need a referral to see the eye doctor? Could my child have a hearing issue if they turn the volume up high on their tablet or TV?

Routine vision and hearing tests are recommended by AAP starting at the age of 4. In rare cases, such as premature children, low birth weight babies, NICU stay for more than 5 days, intubation or incubator interventions, your newborn will require an eye exam prior to nursery discharge. In full-term babies, vision tests are not routinely recommended before 4 years of age; yet, your pediatrician will examine the red reflexes (when light passes through the pupil and reflects off of the retina, like when the eyes appear red in some photos), the external orbits, cornea, retina, and upper and lower eyelids. Amblyopia is the most common cause of vision impairment in children, accounting for 1 to 4% of children's vision impairments, as a result of refractive error in one or both eyes not corrected in early childhood.

Your pediatrician will also ask if your child has excessive tearing, if they are squinting or rubbing their eyes, experiencing photophobia (abnormal light sensitivity), or bumping into objects like doors or walls. Other cues demanding urgent eye doctor referrals are eye deviation or abnormal head posturing (tilting of the head). Strabismus, caused by eye misalignment, is another common reason for ophthalmology referral.

Allen test charts are used in preschool children. They will stand 10 feet away from the vision chart and cover one eye at a time, followed by uncovering both eyes to check the vision in each eye separately and both eyes working together. Allen test cards use figures and pictures. A Snellen eye chart with numbers or letters is used for children 5 and older. Vision function abnormalities could be part of systemic illnesses, genetic, and/or neurodevelopmental syndromes.

Open globe trauma (a puncture or tearing injury to the eye) from paintball guns or BB guns and sharp objects can cause permanent vision loss and blindness. Chemical burns from alkali and acids are other common injuries leading to blindness. Rarely, infections like gonococcal keratoconjunctivitis in the newborn can lead to vision loss. Glaucoma, a disease that can cause vision loss due to damage of the ocular nerve, is hereditary but less frequently seen in children. Hyphema or blood collection in the anterior chamber of the eye after blunt facial trauma can also lead to permanent vision loss.

Hearing tests are also performed routinely, starting at the age of 4. A hearing deficit could be caused by an obstruction between the outer ear and the middle or inner ear interrupting the sound conduction. In children, the most common cause for conductive hearing loss are cerumen impaction (wax build-up) and/or ear infections. In cases of anatomical defects like aural atresia (lack of patent ear canal), the sound conduction is completely blocked.

Sensorineural hearing deficit is the second form of hearing loss resulting from damage or diseases of the inner ear and or the auditory nerve, cranial nerve VIII.

Mixed forms of conductive and sensorineural hearing losses could also be seen.

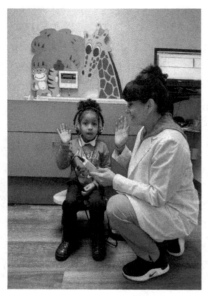
Child in Dr. Daniela's Office
Taking a Vision Test

Less common causes of hearing loss are trauma, tumors, or perforation of the tympanic membranes.

Your doctor will perform audiometry studies, where a series of tones will be sent to the headphones. The pitch and loudness of the tones will be changed, and your child will be asked to raise their hands when they hear the tones.

The Otoacoustic Emission (OAE) Test is more suitable for infants and newborns or children with neurodevelopmental delays preventing them from cooperating with the test. Small probes are inserted in the ear canal, and sound will be sent to the probes. The OAE test cannot tell the difference between conductive and sensorineural. In cases of sensorineural hearing deficits, the ENT doctor and neurologist will decide what your child will need to

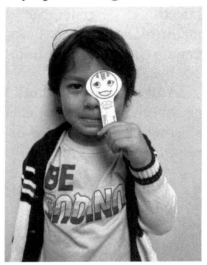

Child in Dr. Daniela's Office Taking a Hearing Test

help them hear: assisting hearing aid devices or a cochlear implant. Early detection and treatment are key. Deafness could be inherited, but because in about 80% of these cases are inherited in an autosomal recessive pattern, they could be left unrecognized until after the child presents with speech delay. About 15% of hearing loss cases are due to genes inherited from a parent who is deaf, and some could be a result of mutations or mitochondrial lineage. Trauma, congenital infections, genetic syndromes, ototoxic medications, and antibiotics used after birth, are among some of the additional causes for deafness.

AAP requires that both vision and hearing tests are offered routinely at each annual well child visit starting at the age of 4 or sooner if concerns are raised by the parents.

94. Why is my child's epilepsy getting worse?

Epilepsy is used as the "umbrella" of diagnoses that include various forms of seizures, but in medical literature, epilepsy is defined as recurrent (more than one) seizures unprovoked by fever. Seizures are the result of abnormal, excessive discharge of the brain's neurons. Seizures can present in different forms, and it is up to the pediatrician to make the primary diagnosis and refer the child to the neurologist for further evaluation and treatment.

The newborn brain varies from the brain of an older child, teens, and adults. The brain of a child from the age of 0–5 years is still immature and developing. This is one of the reasons febrile seizures (those triggered by fever) are so common in this age group. High fever triggers excessive and synchronous discharge of the neurons, presented commonly as convulsions and deviation of the eyes. Parents have difficulties differentiating shivering and chills from febrile seizures and they will run into the clinic or ER, panicking. A short video recording would help in recurrent cases, but in times of emergency, the priority is on keeping the child safe and arranging immediate evaluation and care.

Seizures are also described as "convulsions," which is a term for uncontrollable shaking with the muscles contracting and relaxing rapidly. Drooling or frothing at the mouth, grunting and snoring, loss of bladder or bowel control, sudden falling, teeth clenching, temporary cessation in breathing, and eye movement to the sides are all symptoms of seizures. Sudden falls and unexpected seizures cause a lot of stress for the parents. It creates anxiety and fear.

24/7 supervision is required for young children with seizures. A form with a detailed explanation about how to use their medication with an emergency plan needs to be presented to the school and to all those who are supervising after-school activities. Parents are not supposed to leave their children unsupervised while swimming, bathing, or showering. A helmet is provided for children with atonic seizures (which is a sudden loss of muscle strength followed by a fall.)

Parents and pediatricians should ensure compliance with neurology appointments. Your pediatrician will monitor the child's condition to ensure that they are taking the right amount of medication to control the seizures.

95. How can I best care for my child, who has a rare genetic or chromosomal disorder?

Taking care of a disabled child is physically and emotionally exhausting for the whole family.

Coping with the fact that you have a child with special needs—the extra care, school, transportation, and doctor's appointments—sometimes forces one of the parents to stay home. The siblings are also affected because most of the time is usually devoted to the special child's needs. It is extremely difficult to navigate through the daily struggles, enjoy time with your partner, and have a fulfilling life.

I have seen families fall apart and mothers who were left all alone with their children without financial help other than government assistance. I am very empathetic toward such parents. In an effort to give them my best, I try to spend as much extra time as possible with them, as well as referring them to social workers, psychologists, geneticists, and home care services.

I have been so pleased to live in a city like New York where the state provides excellent care with all supportive services, including home care nurses and medical assistance, special daycares, and schools. But what about the millions of disabled kids all around the world? There are so many factors affecting the care of these children, including the family support and dynamics, the country you live in, the health insurance, and the services that are available.

The first step is always to talk to your pediatrician, who will initiate the process of full evaluation and social services. I often encourage my parents to try an experimental treatment like stem cell therapy or get involved in clinical trials of gene therapies. There are lots of resources and clinics around the world that do have ongoing research programs for children with rare genetic disorders. Caring for a special child is a lifelong process that requires plenty of patience, but with the right direction and support from your doctors and care team, anything is possible. I always try to keep the hopes of my parents and children with special needs high.

It is important to help the parents accept the fact that genetic or chromosomal disorders are not a death sentence. Every one of us has encountered at some point in our lives a smiling, cute child with an extra copy of chromosome 21, called trisomy 21 or Down syndrome. It is the most common genetic

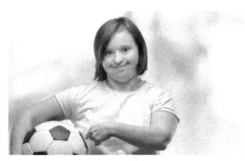

Child with Down Syndrome Playing Soccer

disorder causing intellectual delays, but kids who have Down syndrome are still able to have a fulfilling life and pursue their dreams by competing in sports, graduating from college, and even becoming actors and influencers. There is always hope and with the support of parents, caregivers, teachers, and doctors. Today we are able to provide a meaningful existence to many children with rare and not-so-rare genetic diseases and syndromes.

96.   Is it safe to give my child who is on the autism spectrum anesthesia prior to dental procedures?

Dental care is important for everyone and is part of our daily hygiene. It is difficult to restrain a non-verbal child for surgical or dental procedures. If there is a medical necessity to intervene in the oral cavity and take care of dental needs, then an anesthetic can be the only safe option in non-cooperative children.

Some dentists specialize in the care of children with disabilities or who are on the autism spectrum. I would recommend you first search for them before you approach any other general dentist. A consultation with the anesthesiologist is mandated prior to the procedure. The right medication and method of putting your child to sleep (general anesthesia) will be chosen. Your pediatrician will also examine and medically clear your child 3 to 5 days prior to the procedure. Once it is determined that general anesthesia is safe for your child, the procedure will be scheduled. It is an uncomfortable experience for both parents and child, but with careful preparation and education, dental care for children with special needs can be transformed into a smooth process with great results.

97. How can I help my child with emotional disturbances and depression control their anger?

Statistically, the diagnosed cases of depression and mental illnesses in children are trending up. Perhaps this is also due to preventive medicine. Depression in children younger than 5 years old isn't common, but when a child that young does have depression, it can be difficult to recognize due to its subtle presentation. For toddlers and preschoolers, it is not typical to be withdrawn, have sleep disturbances, decreased or excessive appetites, stay alone in the corner, and not smile or show emotions during fun activities.

Usually my first question for the parents is about recent stressors in the family or the life of the child to help determine the possibility of depression and/or emotional disturbances. For parents, understanding the difference between having an imaginary friend versus hearing voices (for instance that "tell" the child what to do) is key in the diagnosis of schizophrenia, for example.

Both depression and schizophrenia tend to peak during teen years. But letting mental illnesses remain underdiagnosed at an early age (despite behavioral cues) could be detrimental to the future health of the child. Unfortunately, in many countries around the world, talking about mental health is still taboo, and not being able to break the cultural stigma hurts many innocent young lives.

The sooner a psychologist and psychiatrist are involved, the better possibility of a good outcome and brighter future for the child. In the United States, 1 in 6 children age 2–8 years (17.4%) are diagnosed with mental, behavioral, or developmental disorders. For preschoolers and kindergarteners who are at risk for mental illness, their pediatrician will ask them to draw their feelings to determine if they are depressed. Unusual irritability, terrible tantrums, impulsiveness, loss of appetite or obsession with food, and a lack of joy during outdoors activities or playing games are all worrisome signs for a child in the age range of 3–5 years.

In the United States, we also have a depression questionnaire called PHQ 9 (patient health

272

questionnaire 9) which is offered to all patients starting from the age of 12 at every visit to their pediatrician, regardless of whether they show depression symptoms.

The mental health of young children is in the hands of their parents, teachers, and pediatricians. The goal of the therapy is to help change the problematic behaviors, teach them how to cope with the depressive symptoms, improve their social skills, increase self-confidence by

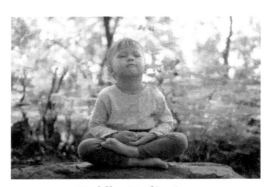

Toddler Meditating

engaging them in sports and other extracurricular activities, adhere to treatment (not necessarily medicated therapy, but cognitive behavioral therapy and play therapy), and prevent the onset of depressive episodes.

I like introducing my little patients and their parents to yoga, pranayama breathing techniques, and meditation. Encouraging them to create rituals in the morning with a 5-minute meditation together with their child to prepare them for the day is a great start. Having a family dinner, followed by walking the dog and sharing the day's experiences, is an amazing way of connecting with your child and learning about their inner world. Having them followed through telehealth visits and sometimes organizing zoom yoga sessions for the child and the parent with my active participation is something I have been integrating into my practice lately.

CHAPTER NINE: KEEPING YOUR YOUNG CHILD SAFE

Dr. Shellie's Mom Memories of Keeping her Children Safe

On my hands and knees, I was crawling around on the floor of my living room, kitchen, and most of the rooms on the first floor of my house. Would I have looked a little bonkers if someone saw this? Absolutely. Yet, it was very important to me to really get a view of possible dangers from my child's perspective and visual viewpoint. I was looking at electrical sockets and making sure there was nothing small on the floor that could go in a mouth. I was seeing where there were sharp edges on furniture and what little hands could get into as soon as I turned my back.

As I found potential hazards for my baby, I added them to a master babyproofing list. I knew that my baby was going to be mobile soon and this was the best way I could think of to make sure I could be proactive with baby proofing.

Of course, you want to keep your child safe, so be proactive in your approach, knowing that little ones must be watched and protected as much as you can in and out of your home. Accidents will happen, but we can plan to keep our children as safe as possible!

Dr. Daniela's Pediatric Prescription for Keeping Children Safe

98. What should I do if my child is allergic to our pet? Is it safe to send my child to preschool if they are allergic to a lot of foods?

Food, animal, and environmental allergies are more frequently observed in urban areas. Most common food allergies, like eggs, cow milk, soy, and wheat peak around 1 year of age and may slowly be outgrown. It could be difficult to differentiate true food allergies from food sensitivities in the first two years of life, and regardless of the atopic triggers, most of them are overgrown during the childhood and adolescent years. On the other hand, peanut, tree nut, and animal allergies tend to last throughout life and can even show up later in adulthood.

With the introduction of solid foods to babies, parents should be warned to watch for symptoms like rashes (called hives), vomiting, and/or loose stool. These are some of the most frequent allergic symptoms in this age group. A very common presentation of multiple food allergies in the first two years of life is atopic dermatitis or eczema. I advise my parents to make a list of all foods that the child reacts to and avoid them for 2–3 months before they slowly reintroduce them later on.

For allergies with severe anaphylactic reactions—requiring an ER visit, epinephrine/EpiPen injection, and oral steroids—complete avoidance of the triggers is mandated. "Anaphylaxis" is the term used to diagnose a severe allergic reaction that occurs within seconds or minutes of exposure to the allergen. Swelling of the lips and face, difficulty breathing, wheezing and choking, hives not sparing the face, low blood pressure, dizziness and fainting, nausea, vomiting, and diarrhea are the predominant symptoms of anaphylaxis. Parents of children requiring epinephrine injection will be educated on when and how to use it, the school will be informed by a signed formal consent and a form with specific instructions and parents should always carry the

EpiPen injection (they come in a pack of 2) with them; keep one in the house and one in the child's daycare or school. During travel or outdoor activities, the EpiPen must be carried by the parent.

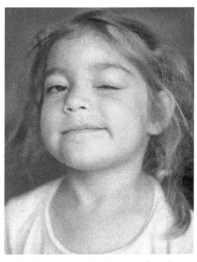

Child in Anaphylactic Shock, a Severe Allergic Reaction

Today, we have two main ways of diagnosing allergies. The first is by testing the blood for Immunoglobulin E (IGE) antibodies formed in response to the allergens and the second is through skin allergy testing. Both are accurate, and most allergy cases are easily handled by the primary pediatrician. The blood test can also show the severity of the allergies, and if the food can be consumed in raw condition or if it is safe only if heated and cooked.

The blood tests also give us information if the child is a candidate for desensitization, especially true for peanut allergies, which are among the most common and could be lethal. Desensitization used for peanut allergies, also known as "peanut allergy immunotherapy," is believed to build a tolerance to peanuts by slowly introducing small amounts until a maximum threshold dose is reached. This is not a cure, but a treatment that minimizes peanut allergic reactions and reduces life-threatening anaphylactic episodes. This treatment must be done only under the supervision of a doctor in a clinical setting.

Going to school is safe when all precautions are being taken, and the child should be taught how to recognize the initial allergic symptoms so they can ask for help.

When it comes to animal allergies, having a hypoallergenic dog or cat is the best way to go, though not always a guarantee. Having the pet for a few weeks before fully committing to adoption or purchase would be less traumatic for the child in case they present with allergies. Hives, sneezing, and allergic conjunctivitis are the usual symptoms.

Talk to your child and explain to them what the risks are if they are old enough to comprehend. If you already happen to live with a pet and your infant or toddler experiences allergic symptoms, it will be wiser to discuss it with your pediatrician. If the severity is mild, it is possible (but not probable) that the child will outgrow it. Not allowing the pets to sleep in the child's room, bathing them more often, and vacuuming the dander daily will be helpful. In general, studies show that growing up with a cat and/or dog lowers the risk of sensitization to an array of allergens. The presence of particular microbes on the dogs and cats protect against developing allergies by diversifying the bacteria in the gastrointestinal tract of babies in the house.

99. When can I start using sunscreen on my child? Is it safe to use spray?

Every parent fantasizes about taking a stroll in the park with their newborn. It is safe to go out as soon as your child is born if the weather permits. Avoiding public places in the first two months of life is advisable. Parents who have more outdoorsy lifestyles frequently ask questions about the right time to start applying sunscreen, using insect repellents, wearing proper clothing, and preventing insect bites. For most babies and children, sunscreen products are approved for use after 6 months of age. I highly advise my parents to use zinc oxide based sunscreens applied 20 minutes before going out to allow for the screen (lotion or stick) to absorb in the skin and get activated. Avoid using sunscreen sprays, as they can be accidentally inhaled or injure the eyes if sprayed on the face. Pay attention to the ingredients of the sunscreen products.

There is a common conception that it's better to wear white or lighter colors on sunny days because black absorbs the sunlight, and therefore makes us hotter, and white reflects the sun and keeps us cool—but this is not exactly the case. Per the Skin Cancer Foundation,[3] it's actually better to wear

---

[3] https://www.skincancer.org/skin-cancer-prevention/sun-protection/sun-protective-clothing/#:~:text=Unbleached%20cotton%20contains%20n

dark or bright colors, because they do a better job of absorbing UV rays and thus minimizing UVA exposure to the skin. So, darker clothes can actually be a better choice, but there are several other points to keep in mind when it comes to choice of fabric.

Factors that contribute to the UPF (the amount of UV radiation that penetrates the skin) rating in fabrics include:

- Composition of the fabric: Unbleached cotton, lightweight silk, and shiny polyester are example of fabrics that reflect radiation well
- Tightness of the knit: The tighter and denser the fabric is, the higher the UPF
- Color: Darker-colored clothes have a higher UPF rating than light-colored clothes
- Stretch: More stretch lowers the UPF rating

---

atural%20lignins,some%20penetration%20from%20UV%20rays

- Moisture: Many fabrics have lower UPF ratings when wet
- Condition: Worn and faded garments reduce the UPF rating
- Coverage: More is better.
- Finishing: Some fabrics are treated with UV-absorbing chemicals

Long sleeves, hats, and sunglasses for older children are all of great help. Use an SPF of 30–50 and an SPF of 30 for daily use. Reapply sunscreen every 3 hours and after each water exposure if it's not water-resistant sunscreen.

My tips for the amount of sunscreen to use:

- 1 teaspoon to the face and neck (don't forget the earlobes, back of the neck, and nose)
- 2 teaspoons to the chest, abdomen, and back
- 1 teaspoon to each upper extremity (arms and hands)
- 2 teaspoons to each lower extremity (legs and feet)

- Avoid sun exposure during the peak hours (from 10 a.m. to 4 p.m.)

Children with light skin are at higher risk of burning. Other high-risk factors for sunburns come from living or traveling close to the equator and to higher-altitude places (including skiing during the winter), or using certain medications like non-steroidal anti-inflammatory drugs (NSAIDS), Motrin, tetracyclines, and antifungal medications.

100. How safe is it to use insect repellent on my child? What should I do if my child gets bitten by a tick?

Insect repellents with a DEET concentration of 10–30% are safe for children and can be used at two months and older. Be aware and read the labels and instructions on the product. Do not use a combination of sunscreen and insect repellent because it does not have the same efficiency. If hiking in areas where ticks are prevalent, using brighter clothing and inspecting the body and scalp of the child during bath time after coming home is an absolute necessity. Brighter clothing will help you spot a potential tick. Placing the dry clothes in dryers on high heat for short periods of time after being outdoors can eliminate potential ticks or insects attached to them.

If you see a tick and you are able to remove it, do so immediately and consult with your pediatrician. If the tick was left in the skin for more than

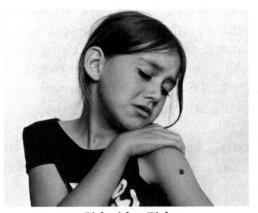

Girl with a Tick

72 hours, preventive oral antibiotics will be prescribed to your child. If you happen to successfully remove the tick, keep it in a plastic bag, and let your pediatrician send it to the lab for review. Use clean, fine-tipped tweezers to grasp the tick, pull upward, but don't twist it, to avoid

leaving parts of the tick in the skin. Remove it gently. Never crush a tick with your fingers.

Avoid myths like using petroleum jelly and nail polish, or using heat to make it detach from the skin. Your goal is to remove the tick as quickly as possible—do not wait for it to detach.

101. Can my child use a walker with wheels to start walking? Can my toddler use a tricycle, scooter, or bike?

Unintentional falls are the leading cause of nonfatal injury in children and account for 8% of fatal children's injuries worldwide. An estimated 230,676 children under 15 months of age were treated for infant walker related injuries in U.S. emergency departments between 1990–2014 (Sims et al., 2018).

Most walker-related injuries are caused by falling down stairs or falling out of the walker. Walkers also provide close proximity to hot beverages, sharp objects, and furniture edges, hence making them very dangerous. Even if the parents are supervising the child, they likely won't be able to react quickly enough to prevent the injury. Stationary activity centers are preferred and recommended by the AAP.

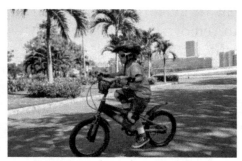

Child Wearing Helmet and Pads Riding a Bike

Most children are introduced to tricycles, bicycles, and scooters at the appropriate age, but many parents are still negligent in the use of safety equipment, like helmets and knee and elbow pads. Children should wear a helmet every single time they use moving vehicles AND be supervised by a responsible adult. Choosing the right size helmet and replacing it as they outgrow it is extremely important, and I always reinforce this fact during my annual prevention visits.

102. When is the best time to childproof my house?

As soon as a child starts crawling and is able to move from place A to B, parents should childproof the house. Pica (a condition where the child eats non-food items) in children ages 6 months to 2 years is common. Infants and toddlers are exploring and instinctively putting everything in their mouths, including toilet paper, coins, batteries, toy pieces, medications, and liquids.

The CDC mandates a CBC (complete blood count) and lead levels blood testing at the ages of 1 and 2 years old. Pica puts your child at risk for iron deficiency anemia and/or lead intoxication.

It is the parent's responsibility to create a safe environment for their infants and toddlers. As pediatricians, it is our task to warn, educate, and advise to keep our little patients happy, healthy, and safe. It is always easier to invest time and money in preventing an injury or accident than treating it after the fact. I often hear my parents saying, "It's ok; I am always supervising my child."

I am sure that you are, but there is no harm in taking precautions.

Parents can feel that their children are immune to accidents and incidents, underestimating the serious complications such events can lead to. I like to post short educational videos on social media, talk about injury prevention during their annual visits, send mass email message reminders, encouraging parents to ask and fill in questionnaires about safety. At times I feel as if I am parenting thousands of kids by being a pediatrician, and I don't mind supportively helping to "parent" more kids around the globe by sharing my knowledge and expertise.

103. Is it safe for my child to ride the school bus? How can I protect my child from bullying at school? Is it safe to send my preschooler with a heavy backpack?

These are common questions and parents like to search for answers by participating in parent support groups on social media. Some parents are overprotective, others extremely anxious and not trustworthy, fearing that the bus driver is not professional enough, or worrying about car accidents. It is a personal choice; whatever makes you comfortable is the right answer. If your child needs to take a school bus, get to know the driver, check their background and experience, inspect the bus, assist your child with taking their seat, and seatbelt them, if possible.

Bullying is another major concern for parents that has gained more attention lately in social media and the school classrooms. Being open with your child and balancing authority with friendship, making them share with you is the best way to find out if your child is at risk for bullying or being bullied. Being in close contact with the school, actively participating in meetings that parents can attend, and scheduling parent-teacher conferences is also something every parent should do. If the bullying persists, consider all options: changing schools, engaging the school psychologist and counselors, and discussing the possibility of consulting a psychotherapist.

Heavy backpacks are another common concern of parents. My best advice to them is to purchase a second set of school books to use at home (check for second-hand books online) and leave their new ones in school. Wearing their backpacks on both shoulders will help with the posture and prevent back pain.

CHAPTER TEN: TRAVELING WITH CHILDREN

Dr. Shellie's Mom Memories of Traveling with Her Children

Traveling with babies and toddlers takes more planning, preparation, and patience than traveling with older children or just adults. However, it can happen peacefully and be fun if you plan it out proactively.

Christine Furman, CEO and founder of Momspiration412 Worldwide and EduPlay Learning, gave us these tips for traveling with children:

- *Make a checklist for what you need to pack and create an agenda for what you will do with the children when you arrive at your destination.*

- *Have the child choose and pack a favorite stuffed animal or toy in their special bag.*
- *Pack snacks for younger kids or bottles for babies.*
- *Pack an extra bag with wipes, hand sanitizer, sunscreen, a change of outfit, and a set of pajamas.*
- *Pack specific entertaining toys that soothe for their age level (e.g., teether for baby cutting teeth and books or tablets for stories for toddlers).*
- *Play games to engage the children with the environment around them such as I Spy.*
- *Road Trip Tip: Ensure that you take many breaks on long drives.*
- *Airplane Tip: Make sure that you have something they can suck on like a lollipop for their ears to stop popping.*
- *Extended Stay Tip: You may want to mail a box with the baby or toddler's things ahead of you so your hands aren't full if you aren't traveling by car.*

I traveled multiple times with my children throughout the years. The moments that were created were priceless.

This chapter has great trips for traveling including vaccine questions for traveling abroad and how to prevent motion sickness. Enjoy the trip and make sure you capture the good moments with photographs to preserve your memories.

Dr. Daniela's Pediatric Prescription for Travel with Children

104. How can we prevent and treat motion sickness?

Motion sickness is a physiological form of dizziness, and it is perfectly normal to experience at any age. However, females are more susceptible, and children less than 2 years old are usually immune to it. Typically, motion sickness is most prevalent at around age 9, and it slowly subsides with age. Motion sickness was first described by Hippocrates. It occurred during boat travel, and the main symptom, nausea, is derived from the Greek word for "ship" (*naus*). The most common type is sea sickness, and it is induced by the low-frequency motion of the boat.

How to Prevent Motion Sickness

- Look at the horizon at a stationary object.

- Avoid reading or looking at a screen while in a moving environment.
- Select seats where the motion of the vehicle will be felt the least, such as the middle of the boat or car.

How to Treat Motion Sickness

- Give your child antihistamines like Benadryl or the anticholinergic drug Scopolamine only after you discuss it and if recommended by your pediatrician. They come in different forms, syrup, chewable tablets, transdermal patches, sublingual (under the tongue), buccal (kept inside the mouth close to the cheeks), and rectal.
- Give your child ginger candy to chew or suck on.
- Provide your child with an acupressure band to wear around the wrist.

105. Can I travel to countries that are at high risk of measles, mumps, and rubella if my child hasn't been vaccinated for them?

Vaccines and travel are handled either by general pediatricians or travel clinics. Every country has specific recommendations for entrance, and without fulfilling the requirements, travelers won't be able to cross the borders of the destination country.

MMR is a live vaccine developed to provide immunity against 3 viral illnesses. "MMR" stands for "measles, mumps, and rubella," which are common in countries where the rates of immunizations are low, or the immunization protocol does not require MMR vaccination. These tend to be countries that rely on natural immunity created by contracting the disease and building up natural antibodies.

In the United States and most other countries, the MMR vaccine is administered at 1 year of age followed by a booster shot at 4 years. There are differences in vaccine production based on manufacturers around the globe. In some places, it is given as separate components, but in the United States, it is given as one combination vaccine.

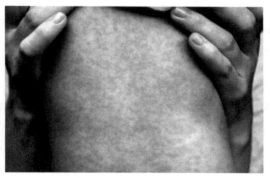

Measles Rash on Baby's Chest

If your child is headed to a place with a high risk of MMR and is under the age of 1 year, they will be immunized at 6 months of age at the earliest, but they will require a third dose since they will still be receiving their 1- and 4-year-old shots. If your child is 12 months old, they will require 2 doses of MMR spread 28 days apart.

Today, measles are extremely rare and preventable, but if acquired, it causes the following symptoms: high fever, flu-like symptoms with severe respiratory symptoms like hacking cough and runny nose, conjunctivitis, and fatigue.

The measles rash appears 2–3 days after the fever. The infected person is contagious from about 5 days before the appearance of the rash to about 4 days afterwards. The rash starts spreading from the face down to the trunk and extremities. Something that is a common characteristic of the disease is Koplik's spots that appear after the body rash (these are red spots with a bluish center in the back of the mouth).

People may get infected in public places even without person-to-person contact. The viral illness runs its course unless there are complications that can lead to encephalitis, pneumonia, ear infections, or gastroenteritis.

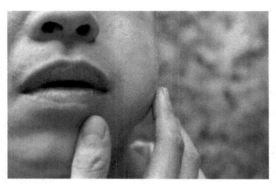
Child with Mumps with Face Swelling

Mumps occurs worldwide, the peak incidence is typically in the late winter to early spring, but outbreaks can occur at any time. It is rare in infants under the age of 1 who have protection from maternal antibodies. The peak is in school-aged children and college-aged young adults. It has less severe presentation and it is also caused by a virus transmitted through air droplets by coughing, sneezing, direct contact, or fomites (objects or materials that are likely to carry infection such as clothes, utensils, and furniture).

Mumps affects the salivary and parotid glands and presents with swelling and pain over the lower part of the jaw. It goes away on its own, unless complicated with oophoritis in females (inflammation of the ovaries, presenting with lower abdominal pain, fever, and vomiting or orchitis in males (testicular pain and swelling) and aseptic meningitis or encephalitis (brain infections). Another rare complication is deafness after an acute and severe presentation of the illness.

Rubella has a characteristic body rash similar to that of measles. It

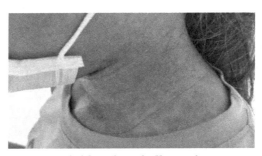

Child with Rubella Rash

presents with fever and respiratory symptoms but should go away on its own. If a pregnant unimmunized woman carries the disease in the first 16 weeks of pregnancy, the child may die *in utero* or have severe complications after birth like a loss of hearing and eyesight, cataracts, glaucoma, heart problems, intellectual disabilities, and liver or spleen damage. Rubella has been declared eradicated in the United States as of 2004, but outbreaks around the world are still reported.

Prevention is the key for all these three viral illnesses. Follow the advice of your pediatrician.

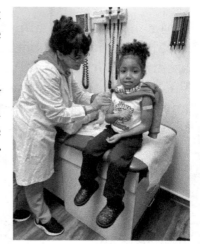

Dr. Daniela's Nurse
Administering Vaccines

106. What tips do you have for traveling abroad with our child?

Traveling with children is not always easy and enjoyable. You need to prepare and pack for yourself and for your children. You must pre-calculate every possible scenario from sickness to injuries. International travel means everything from malaria prevention to making sure all their vaccines are up-to-date.

Togetherness with families during travel makes it more fun, especially when there are new memories to make. Choosing a vacation where the whole family will have fun is important. Pick the best place to explore with your children depending on their age, the facilities, and age-appropriate activities offered at the chosen location and venue. Cruises can be easier to handle and more affordable, but after the Covid-19 pandemic a lot of parents are reluctant to take a chance considering the higher risk of acquiring disease. Amusement parks are outdoorsy and also a common destination.

I like to schedule my patients one week prior to their travel so I can counsel and offer my special "Dr. Daniela's Travel Pack and First Aid Kit" by prescribing some of the most needed medication in case of minor emergencies.

Telemedicine virtual visits give my parents a lot of comfort knowing they can reach me or my colleagues even when they are away from home. One of the most common questions I get prior traveling is, "Doc can you prescribe me antibiotics in case my child gets diarrhea?" And the answer is "no," because the most common cause of traveler's diarrhea is *E. coli* 0157:H7, which, if treated with oral antibiotics, can lead to harmful hemolytic uremic syndrome (Hus) complications, which negatively affects the kidneys. In case of mild gastrointestinal infection, presenting with loose stools accompanied with nausea and vomiting without abdominal pain, bloody stool or fever, you can manage the condition by offering oral hydration and childrens' electrolytes commonly sold in any pharmacy around the world. Kids' probiotics could be beneficial as well. Getting international health insurance for the whole family before your trip is highly recommended and will give you peace of mind.

If the child develops loose but bloody diarrhea, fever, and/or acute abdominal pain with signs of dehydration, they must be brought to the ER for medical evaluation.

Don't forget your sunscreen, insect repellents, and chronic medication if the child is on any. Antipyretics (or fever medication), antihistamines (anti-allergics) for mild allergies, and pain medications should always be carried. Alcohol pads and bandages are always good to have handy. An EpiPen and Benadryl for children with allergies should be packed in a first aid bag. Every case and every child has different needs, and this is why a travel consultation with your pediatrician is always helpful. Bon voyage!

CHAPTER ELEVEN: EMERGENCIES

Dr. Shellie's Mom Memories of Emergencies

Don't panic! That's the number one tip when emergencies happen. As the parent, you need to keep your wits about you. If you end up melting down, it will only make the situation worse. Take a deep breath, analyze the situation, and take immediate steps to de-escalate it. Read this book so if an emergency occurs, you will know what to do.

In this chapter, Dr. Daniela covers the most common emergency situations. You will understand what to do if your child is bitten by a dog or choking on a piece of food. You need to know the common injuries that need immediate medical attention from a professional: severe burns, frostbite, Inflicted puncture wounds, eye injuries, and bone fractures.

We suggest taking a CPR and first aid course through an official organization such as The American Red Cross. Also, be sure that others who provide caregiving, including babysitters, have been certified in this as well.

You need to know when to call 911 in a true emergency, when to drive to the emergency room or urgent care, and when to call the pediatrician. Getting the support and help you need for your child in an emergency situation is vital.

You can handle the emergency. Just be aware and prepared with the knowledge.

Dr. Daniela's Pediatric Prescription for Emergencies

107. What do I do if my child is bitten by an animal?

Dogs are the most loyal friends of humans, but occasionally accidents can happen. Here are my tips on how to handle a dog bite:

1.) Stop the bleeding.

2.) Clean the wound with soap and water.

3.) Proceed to the nearest ER so they can clean the wound. They may administer vaccines and/or tetanus shots.

4.) Call your doctor.

If the dog is domesticated (someone's pet) and is known to be healthy and fully-immunized and can be observed for 10 days, there is no need for rabies immunoglobulin and a rabies vaccine for the child who was bitten.

If it's an unknown street dog that runs away and can't be observed for 10 days, then rabies immunoglobulin and a tetanus shot are required. If the

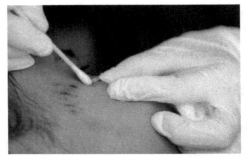

Child with a Dog Bite Wound on the Face

skin is punctured, then an antibiotic against *Pasteurella multocida* (oral flora of the dog) is needed. There should be no suturing or closure of the laceration or wound unless it is affecting the face.

Other animals that carry rabies are racoons, skunks, bats, and foxes. Often after a dog bite or any animal bite at an early age, the child is at risk of suffering post-traumatic stress disorder (PTSD) for the rest of their lives, so such accidents can't be taken lightly. Referral to a psychologist is warranted, especially if the child shows signs of

PTSD like night terrors, fear of going outside or playing in the park, irritability, and phobia of dogs.

108. What do I do if my child is in an accident, such as in a car, a bicycle, tricycle, scooter, or skiing?

Accidents happen. Do your best as a caretaker and parent to prevent, prevent, and prevent! Do not wait for the moment you leave the nursery with a newborn. Do your research, and then purchase and install the car seat. Make sure it is the right size for your newborn, and carefully read the manufacturer's instructions. For the first 2 years of life, the position of your child in a car seat will be rear-facing, and then all you need to do is buy the appropriate car seat based on weight and age and follow the instructions. When the child reaches the age for a car seat booster, assist them and seat belt them before you take the wheel.

Tricycles, bicycles, and scooters all need the appropriate equipment. Helmets and knee and elbow support pads will protect your child from harmful and sometimes lethal injuries. Skiing is a great winter sport that also mandates helmets and warm clothing. Supervision and safety equipment are important for helping to prevent injuries.

If the accident results in head trauma with loss of consciousness, major bleeding, and/or bone deformities, call emergency medical services to get help immediately.

Tooth injuries are seen in 50% of children under the age of 5, and the percentage could be even higher because most of them remained unreported. Tooth damage can occur in relation to head or neck trauma during falls or bike, scooter, and motor vehicle accidents. The most commonly injured teeth are the front top and bottom teeth. If a primary (baby) tooth has been knocked out, do not attempt to place it back in the socket. We want to protect the permanent tooth's bud.

Knocking out a permanent tooth, though, is a true emergency. Allowing the tooth to be exposed to air for more than 15 minutes will dry out the periodontal ligament and could prevent the dentist from successfully reattaching the tooth. Instead, keep the tooth wet, and holding it by the crown (top), try to place it back into the socket. If the socket is bleeding or clotted, attempt to rinse, remove the clot, and place the tooth back in the socket. Then ask your child to bite on a towel or gauze. If you can't get the tooth back into the socket, DO NOT dry it. Put it in a container with cold milk or your child's saliva (just ask them to spit into the container) to store it until you can seek medical help and proceed to the nearest ER or see your dentist if available.

Cold milk storage and saliva can last longer than an hour, but you should meet with your dentist immediately, if possible. An emergency tooth preserving system called "Save a tooth" could be purchased and kept in the house ahead of time, in case of such an accident. It is the only FDA-approved media nourishing the tooth for up to 24 hours and having a 90% success rate for reimplantation.

Do not let your child keep the avulsed tooth in their mouth as they can damage, swallow and even aspirate it which is another medical emergency.

109. How do I deal with emergencies like eye injuries and fractures?

In the summers, in pediatric emergency rooms, we see overwhelming cases of fractures, and most of them are inflicted by falls from monkey bars, motor vehicle accidents (MVAs), scooters, and bike accidents. The playgrounds in most countries today have padded and soft ground, but in some less-developed countries, they are still cemented and dangerously constructed. Regardless of the ground surface, there are still many falls, and some involve head and neck trauma with episodes of loss of consciousness, others result in severe but rarely open fractures of the extremities. Call the ambulance if any of the above occurs.

Seatbelt injuries during MVAs are not uncommon, and even with side-door airbags, contusions (bruising) are often seen. Blunt trauma to the abdomen from the belt compressing the abdominal wall during the car accident and injuring the solid abdominal organs (usually the spleen and liver) are common. Look for signs of bruising where the seatbelt rests across the belly.

316

Eye injuries often happen in toddlers and young children from spraying their eyes with perfumes,

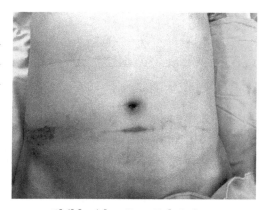

Child with a Seat Belt Injury

deodorants, Windex, or other home cleaning products. Having eyes poked with sharp objects like pencils, branches of trees, scissors, knives, thorns, and writing instruments, sometimes by older siblings, is not uncommon. Eyeball injuries suffered during ball sports, motor vehicle collisions or fights are also seen, but these are more often in the adolescent age group.

After an accident has occurred, the parent's role is to keep the child safe while waiting for the ambulance to arrive. Once in the ER, the patient will be stabilized, vital signs will be assessed, and immediate professional care will be provided for your child.

110. What should I do if my child is choking?

Choking is a medical emergency. Anatomic abnormalities are some of the reasons behind choking and asphyxia in the first hours or days of life. Regardless of the reason (e.g., tracheoesophageal fistula TEF, laryngotracheal cleft (LTEC), airway obstructions, or neurological causes), there is disruption of the coordination of swallowing and breathing. Choking during breastfeeding or formula feeding can happen if the parents are not keeping their children in the correct position and the child is latching too fast or using the wrong size bottle.

Latching specialists are always available in the hospital nursery and they work closely with the parents to educate them on the proper breastfeeding techniques. Hiccups are commonly seen during feedings, and parents must interrupt the feedings while keeping the infant in an upright position, burping them, and resuming the feedings only after the hiccups have resolved.

Hiccups happen when the child is latching too fast, is overfed, or swallows lots of gas during feedings. The expanded stomach pushes against the diaphragm and causes a spasm that is followed by a sudden inspiration that ends with the closure of the glottis (the opening between the vocal cords), generating the "hic" sound, known as a hiccup.

Putting your child in a car seat or overfeeding them without allowing time for them to burp and digest could trigger spitting up followed by choking. Either of these scenarios can also complicate physiological GERD (gastroesophageal reflux disease—acid reflux that happens with each feeding—with choking.

An acute life-threatening event (ALTE) can also present as choking. ALTE is not a specific diagnosis, but rather a chief complaint where the child needs immediate medical attention, which may interrupt breathing.

Toddlers who are prone to pica (a condition where they eat or crave things that are not edible) and can choke on foreign bodies like toy pieces, coins, and batteries.

The foods most commonly regarded as choking hazards are candy, tree nuts, grapes, carrots, cherries, and hot dogs. You must be sure that any foods like grapes are cut up small enough to pass through the throat even if it isn't chewed completely.

Feeding a child without supervision with foods that are potential choking hazards must be avoided. All parents should have basic knowledge of how to provide first aid for choking and certify for CPR prior to the baby's birth and refresh their skills every 2 years.

Every annual exam must include counseling on choking and injury prevention. If you see your child choking on something—regardless of whether they lose consciousness—do CPR and 911 call. Follow this with an ER visit and exam.

111. What should I do if my child ingests something toxic?

Another commonly seen accident that requires an ER visit and immediate care is intoxication—when a child is exposed to something that makes them sick from ingestion, inhalation, or touch. If intoxication is witnessed, it is easier to take immediate action and call poison control when you are dealing with a stable and conscious child, but if unwitnessed, the care could be delayed until after the child presents with signs of intoxication.

These are a couple common examples of intoxication and what to do.

- Unintentional ingestion of medications in liquid, solid, or chewable form is seen mostly in the age group of 1 to 5 years. Vitamins, aspirin, diabetes tablets, blood pressure pills, and fever control medications are some of the most commonly ingested medications by children. If you notice that your child successfully opened a medication bottle and is acting not like themselves:

drowsy, fatigued, unresponsive, walking off balance, having difficulty breathing, choking, or vomiting, call an ambulance immediately.

- Carbon monoxide intoxication is easily preventable by installing carbon monoxide detectors. Carbon monoxide (CO) is an odorless, colorless, tasteless, nonirritating gas. When it gets into the bloodstream, the result is an impaired transport of oxygen to the major body organs, which can then shut down quickly.

Symptoms of carbon monoxide intoxication to watch for include:

- Headaches
- Dizziness
- Nausea and vomiting
- Cough and/or choking
- Confusion
- Shortness of breath
- Throat and eye irritation
- Chest tightness

- Mild confusion and weakness, which may quickly manifest with coma

Parents must either call Poison Control if the child is stable or proceed to the nearest ER if the child is lethargic or unresponsive.

When a child is found to be intoxicated, the role of the medical provider is first and foremost to stabilize the

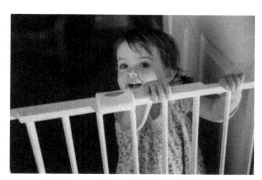
Childproofing with a Baby Gate

airway, breathing, and circulation and then to look for potential reasons for intoxication. Consider what medications or vitamins you have in your house that your child could have ingested to help identify what the child ate so the medical team can act with available antidotes. Bring with you all bottles and medications found next to your child to help the ER doctor with an efficient and quick intervention.

112. What should I do if my child is convulsing?

Convulsions, also known as seizures, are responsible for 1–2% of ER visits in the United States. Seizures could be benign when provoked by fever. Parents fear that their children may die from the seizure, so they then worry about their child getting another febrile cold—a cold that presents with a fever. Febrile seizures (FS)—seizures set off by a fever—have a rate in Western populations of 2.4% and are statistically higher in Japanese populations. One in 3 children with FS will have further episodes between 6 months and 6 years of age. The overall sibling risk is 8%, compared with the population risk of 2.4%. Children with FS have 3–6 times the increased risk of developing epilepsy (Hammans, 2009).

The classification and differential diagnosis of seizures is broad and complicated. Seizures are intermittent, go away on their own, and are the result of excessive discharge of neurons.

Epilepsy is diagnosed when there are at least two unprovoked seizures occurring more than 24 hours apart. Other diagnostic factors include underlying conditions like stroke, central nervous system infection, traumatic brain injury, or genetic disorders. These can increase the probability of future occurrences of seizures.

The first seizure witnessed by parents is undeniably a terrifying experience. Most seizures have full clinical presentation with convulsions, deviation of the eyes, and unresponsiveness, but there is a group of seizures presenting more subtly (minimal clinical expression). They involve spacing out or staring at one spot or object without responding when the child's name is called, known as "absence seizures."

Regardless of the cause, when a seizure occurs, the most important action a parent can take is to keep the child safe by turning them on their side and maintaining an open airway without interfering. Keep the child on their side, and ensure the airway is open while calling for help.

Call for an ambulance or ask someone to do it for you.

Do not attempt to pull the tongue out during the convulsions, the child will not swallow their tongue, but you can injure them or get bitten. Loosen their clothes and stay close to the child until help arrives.

Because febrile seizures are most commonly observed in the 0–5 age group, learning how to prevent the seizures by controlling a fever when the child gets one with round-the-clock anti-fever medication and monitoring the child while they have a fever are the best preventive measures.

Instructions on how to administer rectal or nasal diazepam spray in case of future seizures will be given by your pediatrician. Parents of children who have seizures should have the medication at home and during travel and check the expiration date. Counseling and educating the parents, encouraging them to comply with the neurology appointments is of significant importance.

If the parents are well-trained, they will be able to best assist their children in case of emergency before professional medical care arrives. EMS paramedics know how to administer the first line anticonvulsant medications and stabilize the patient's airway, breathing, and circulation. Your child's daycare or school will need a medical form with specific instructions for when and how to administer first line medications in case of a seizure.

In the ER, after the child regains consciousness, a neurology consultation and an electroencephalogram (EEG) will be performed. Blood work will be taken to assure that glucose and all electrolytes are within normal limits. With the first afebrile seizure—not triggered by a fever—brain imaging studies will be considered to rule out structural and anatomical anomalies.

After regaining consciousness from a seizure, your child will be drowsy; there is a postictal phase during which the brain will slowly regain full consciousness. Some of the physical signs of this phase are headaches, loss of bladder or bowel function, nausea, abdominal pain, sore muscles, and feeling extremely weak or faint.

113. What unique health issues should adoptive parents consider?

Adopting a child is a huge decision made by one or two adults who commit to take care of a child who is not biologically theirs.

The U.S. Department of State requires that internationally adopted children undergo a medical examination in their birth country called "panel evaluation" by a U.S. clinician before admission into the United States. The clinical evaluation is limited to screening for physical and mental disorders and certain communicable diseases like syphilis, gonorrhea, tuberculosis, and HIV.

Medical records from their birth country must be included and reviewed. Laboratory testing for syphilis, Hepatitis B, and HIV are routinely available for all countries of adoption. All children should have documented TB testing either through a QuantiFERON blood test (QFT) or a tuberculin skin test. Labs should be done a few weeks to a month prior to admission into the United States (or any other country of entry). All internationally adopted children are examined by their newly assigned pediatrician within 2 weeks of arrival.

As a pediatrician of many adopted children throughout the years, my focus has been on nutritional status. and initial screening for congenital anomalies, (including fetal alcohol syndrome). It's important that the pediatrician doesn't miss signs of sexual or physical abuse, evaluates their hearing and vision, and assesses their oral health and developmental status. Screening for infectious diseases not covered by the blood serological testing prior to arrival is part of the initial well child visit. Blood lead levels, screening for complete blood count (CBC) and iron deficiency anemia, thyroid function testing, and hemoglobin electrophoresis for sickle cell disease are all important labs to consider. Screening for intestinal parasites is also required. Children adopted from malaria endemic regions will require a malaria screening as well. In areas where chagas disease is endemic, a screening will be prompted.

Once you make the decision to adopt, search for a good pediatrician and work collaboratively throughout the entire process of adoption. Best wishes to your family!

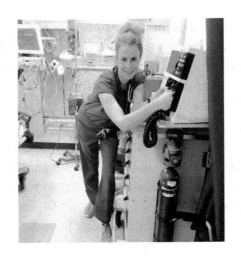

CONCLUSION: YOUR HAPPY, RESILIENT, AND HEALTHY CHILD

The happiness of your child in the first years of life depends on your happiness as a parent. What are the family dynamics? Is the child safe at home? Are the parents caring and loving? Are the parents financially stable? How do they cope with solving problems and how do they face stress and challenges? These are all things that should be considered within the family dynamic while raising a young child.

Families do not look one particular way. From parents with disabilities to a variety of races, religions, cultural backgrounds, and more, families are unique in their structure, beliefs, and ideals. When I started my residency program at Mount Sinai Hospital in Manhattan affiliated with Elmhurst Hospital, Queens, I could not foresee the day when I would be able to stock books in my pediatric clinic's library with titles like *My Two Moms* and *My Two Amazing Dads*. It never mattered to me if my little kiddos had two moms, two dads, or a mom and a dad, were adopted, fostered, or raised by a member of their nuclear or extended families. It is all about living happily and being loved.

We live in an imperfect world. Yet, when we face our challenges with wisdom and maturity we can survive and thrive with our children. Have the courage to ask for help from your mentors, friends, teachers, and pediatricians. You can find balance in your lives and families.

Remember that your child is happy when you are happy!

Your child's resilience is usually learned through exposure and experience. Teach them independence at an early age, and be supportive but not overprotective and controlling. Let them find their passions, which can be more easily said than done. Help them find themselves and be present for them. Love them without reservation, and let them fly freely and happily. You as parents do not have ownership of your children. You are entrusted with their care.

Finding one's passion requires trying lots of different things, through art, dance, sports, chess, and robotic clubs... you name it. Do not attempt to impose or project your unfulfilled dreams and passions on your child. You give them wings to fly so they can someday soar to find themselves and their purpose.

It is your responsibility as a parent to do your best to help this child thrive in life. The health of your child during the beginning years begins with having a safe home and healthy dietary choices; plus, you should offer your child opportunities for exploration, adventure, fun, self-expression, and movement-based activities. You are the guide on the side of your precious little ones as they successfully grow into happy and healthy children.

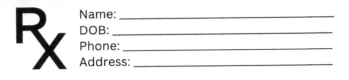

Name: _____
DOB: _____
Phone: _____
Address: _____

The Prescription for a Happy, Resilient, and Healthy Child is:

A loving home that has been child-proofed

Fully stocked first aid kit, carbon monoxide/smoke detector, and fire extinguisher

A great pediatrician seen at 3-5 days after birth, then at 1, 2, 4, 6, 9, 12, 15, 18, 24, 30, 36, and 48 months, and then yearly, and as needed

Healthy, nutritious meals (and snacks and treats as needed)

Unlimited hugs and thirst for learning about the world around them

Rest, sleep, and ample amounts of imaginative fun

Dedicated teachers

Parent(s) who have their hearts full of love

The bestselling book *The Prescription for a Happy and Healthy Child*!

Elligible for Endless Refills ✔

Dr. Shellie Hipsky

About the Authors

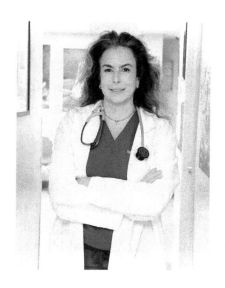

Daniela Atanassova-Lineva, MD

Daniela Atanassova-Lineva, MD, is dedicated to the health of children and families at Peds For Kids in Rego Park, New York. A board-certified pediatrician and a fellow of the Academy of Pediatrics' section of adolescent medicine, she was named among America's top pediatricians for 13 years running. Born in Bulgaria, she showed an interest in medicine at an early age and pursued it with dedication and perseverance.

Dr. Atanassova-Lineva started her elementary education in Kenitra, Morocco, where she attended Lycee Francais. She attended The International School of Foreign Languages for high school and graduated as the valedictorian in her native town of Russe, Bulgaria.

Earning a maximum medical school admittance score, Dr. Atanassova-Lineva won acceptance to Varna Medical University in Bulgaria where she earned her medical degree. Shortly after graduating from Varna Medical University, she led research in neuroscience and child psychiatry. She then completed a pediatric residency at Mount Sinai School of Medicine, affiliated with Elmhurst Hospital in Queens, New York.

She remained an assistant clinical professor in the hospital's Department of Pediatric Emergency Medicine for more than 15 years where she instructed medical students and pediatric residents. Currently she teaches the Stony Brook University physician's assistant students by mentoring them during clinical rotations in pediatrics at her private office. In addition, Dr. Atanassova-Lineva maintains affiliations with the prestigious NorthWell Children's Hospital in Long Island, New York Presbyterian-Queens Hospital, and Mount Sinai Hospital, Manhattan.

Dr. Atanassova-Lineva's areas of clinical interest span emergency medicine, pediatric primary care, and adolescent medicine, as well as asthma, allergic disorders, obesity, nutrition, and dermatology, integrated with aesthetic medicine. As a pediatric specialist, her emphasis remains on prevention for young patients. She received certifications in aesthetic medicine in 2016 and in obesity medicine from Harvard University in 2019.

Dr. Atanassova-Lineva has practiced pediatric and emergency medicine for more than 20 years. As a veteran pediatrician, she has seen how parents' health affects children. Her new focus is extending her practice to encompass treatment for the entire family by offering group counseling and telehealth medicine and remaining in close contact with the parents of her patients, regardless of distance, location, and time zone differences.

Dr. Atanassova-Lineva has published scholarly articles on the subjects of obesity, nutrition, sports medicine, and children with cleft lip and palate.

In 2016 Dr Atanassova-Lineva lost her 20 year old daughter Stefani Lineva (a division 1 tennis player attending a pre-med college program) in a hit-and-run accident. The tragedy inspired her to create a nonprofit in memory of her beloved Stefani, "Stefani Forever 20." Together with her son Daniel, she became the CEO of this organization with the mission to promote tennis to underprivileged children worldwide.

Volunteering has always come naturally to Dr. Atanassova-Lineva, and she has been donating her time helping children in Nepal, India, Nicaragua, Honduras, Panama, El Salvador, Guatemala, and Ecuador.

Fluent in five languages, Dr. Atanassova-Lineva has delivered numerous presentations at the

Eastern European Meetings of Pediatrics and TV presentations on TV5Monde in Paris, France, the Telemundo TV channel in New York, and Bulgarian and Russian Radio Stations. The International Pediatric Association honored Dr. Atanassova-Lineva as a leading physician in the world and top pediatrician in Queens, New York. The following year, she was recognized with a "Patients' Choice Award." In 2018 Dr. Atanassova-Lineva was honored to cut the ribbon on the newly renovated Pediatric Clinic of Gotham Health and Hospital Corporations in Jackson Heights, New York. The International Association of Top Professionals honored Dr. Atanassova-Lineva as the "Top Pediatrician of the Year" for 2022. At the International Business Excellence Awards in 2023, Dr. Atanassova-Lineva was honored with the "Lifetime Achievement in Pediatric Medical Care Award."

Dr. Atanassova-Lineva appeared on the front page of *IAOTP Magazine* in 2022 and in *25 A Magazine*, Long Island, New York, where she published articles about her achievements.

For more information and resources from Dr. Daniela Atanassova-Lineva for raising happy and healthy children please go to Peds4Kids.com. Scan the QR code below to go directly to the site.

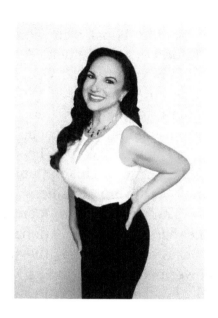

Dr. Shellie Hipsky

Dr. Shellie Hipsky is the CEO of Inspiring Lives International, the executive director of the Global Sisterhood (which helps women and children around the world), and the editor-in-chief of *Inspiring Lives Magazine*. Dr. Shellie Hipsky's doctorate is an Ed.D. in educational leadership from Duquesne University.

The president of the United States of America honored Dr. Shellie Hipsky in 2023 with the Presidential Lifetime Achievement Award for her over 4,000 hours of volunteer service! In 2022, she was heralded as an "Empowered Woman," "Elite Business Leaders to Watch," "Most Influential Female Entrepreneurship Coach," "A Top Entrepreneur in the us," "Women Leaders to Look Up To," "Top 10 Unstoppable Women Entrepreneurs," "Top 20 Business Coaches to Watch For," "The 10 Most Influential Women Business Leaders," and "Global Woman Influencer." She was honored as the world's "Top Global Empowerment Coach" in Las Vegas by the International Association of Top Professionals. In 2023, she was also named IATOP's "Top Inspirational CEO" and at the International Business Excellence Awards she received the "International Visionary Leadership Award."

An award-winning author, she wrote the *Common Threads* trilogy on *Inspiration, Empowerment,* and *Balance* based on her *Empowering Women Radio* show. Her 13th book, *Ball Gowns to Yoga Pants: Entrepreneurial*

Secrets to Create Your Dream Business and Brand, and her newly released 14th book, *Mom Magic Mompreneur: The Magic of Motherhood and how it's Changing the World*, were both international bestsellers in multiple countries.

Dr. Shellie Hipsky was a tenured university undergraduate through doctoral professor. During her former career, she was also a special education teacher, ran a group home for adults on the autism spectrum, and was an assistant principal at a school of children with emotional and behavioral needs.

Active in the world of media, she was the host of both *Empowering Women Radio* and *Inspiring Lives with Dr. Shellie* on NBC. She has keynoted internationally from Passion to Profits in Hollywood to prestigious educational settings such as Harvard, Columbia, Pepperdine, and The University of Oxford in England. She has been featured on over 60 magazine covers and on all the major television networks. She frequently writes for *Forbes* and serves on their expert panel of coaches. Dr. Shellie's podcasts and vocal recording of "And All That Jazz" from the musical *Chicago* can be heard on Spotify and iTunes. Her signature keynote can be seen on Amazon Prime on *Speak Up!* and she recently filmed the docu-series *The Making of an Entrepreneur*.

Often launching businesses for women, her latest business venture is Dr. Shellie's Style Swap which helps women answer the question, "What am I going to wear?"

With her Global Sisterhood 501(c)(3) she collaborates with other charities and performs acts of #PopUpGiving to help women around the world from Pittsburgh to Pakistan who are challenged with issues ranging from domestic violence to homelessness.

Dr. Shellie is currently enrolling women who are experiencing overwhelm with time balance and creating abundance while striving for the next level of their businesses and lives through her signature EmpowerU Master Class and her World Class VIP coaching experiences. Dr. Shellie Hipsky is the Global Empowerment Coach who is inspiring women entrepreneurs and leaders internationally.

RESOURCES

Websites

www.healthychildren.org

www.childmind.org

www.cdc.gov

www.publications.aap.org

Books

American Academy of Pediatrics. (2019). *Caring for Your Baby and Young Child, 7th Edition: Birth to Age 5 Paperback.* AAP.

Ari Brown and Denise Fields (2015). *Baby 411: Clear Answers and Smart Advice for Your Baby's First Year.* Windsor Peak Press.

Cook, W. & Klass, K. (2020). *Mayo Clinic Guide to Your Baby's First Years*. Mayo Clinic Press.

Karp, H. & Fannon, T. (2008). *The Happiest Toddler on the Block: How to Eliminate Tantrums and Raise a Patient, Respectful and Cooperative One- to Four-Year-Old*, Revised Edition. Happiest Baby Inc.

Lieberman, Alicia. (2017). *The Emotional Life of the Toddler*. Simon and Schuster.

 Oster, E. (2020). *Cribsheet: A Data-Driven Guide to Better, More Relaxed Parenting, from Birth to Preschool (The ParentData Series)*. Penguin Press.

INDEX

BIBLIOGRAPHY

Bass, M.M., Duchowny, C.A. & Llabre, M.M. (2009). The Effect of Therapeutic Horseback Riding on Social Functioning in Children with Autism. *J Autism Dev Disord* 39, 1261–1267. https://doi.org/10.1007/s10803-009-0734-3

Bilgin A, Wolke D. Parental use of 'cry it out' in infants: no adverse effects on attachment and behavioural development at 18 months. *J Child Psychol Psychiatry.* 2020 Nov; 61(11):1184-1193. doi: 10.1111/jcpp.13223. Epub 2020 Mar 10. PMID: 32155677.
https://pubmed.ncbi.nlm.nih.gov/32155677/

Moon RY, Tanabe KO, Yang DC, Young HA, Hauck FR. Pacifier use and SIDS: evidence for a consistently reduced risk. *Matern Child Health J.* 2012 Apr;16(3):609-14. doi: 10.1007/s10995-011-0793-x. PMID: 21505778.

Reda SM, El-Ghoneimy DH, Afifi HM. Clinical predictors of primary immunodeficiency diseases in children. *Allergy Asthma Immunol Res.* 2013 Mar;5(2):88-95. doi: 10.4168/aair.2013.5.2.88. Epub 2012 Nov 2. PMID: 23450209; PMCID: PMC3579097.

Sims A, Chounthirath T, Yang J, Hodges NL, Smith GA. (Oct., 2018) Infant Walker-Related Injuries in the United States. *Pediatrics.* 142(4):e20174332. doi: 10.1542/peds.2017-4332. Epub 2018 Sep 17. PMID: 30224365.

Varadhi, A., Hageman, J. R., Yu, K. O. (2013). The 'five fingers' of the diagnostic evaluation for suspected immunodeficiency. *Pediatric Annals, 42*(5), 210-215.

Warner, T.T., Hammans, S.R. (2009). *Practical Guide to Neurogenetics.* Elsevier Health Sciences.

World Health Organization. (June 9, 2021a). Malnutrition. *WHO Fact Sheets.* https://www.who.int/news-room/fact-sheets/detail/malnutrition

World Health Organization. (June 9, 2021b). Obesity and Overweight. *WHO Fact Sheets.* https://www.who.int/news-room/fact-sheets/detail/obesity-and-overweight

CPSIA information can be obtained
at www.ICGtesting.com
Printed in the USA
LVHW052137170623
750085LV00011B/1493